Superstitions Connected with the History and Practice of Medicine and Surgery

by Thomas Joseph Pettigrew

with an introduction by Dahlia V. Nightly

This work contains material that was originally published in 1844.

This publication is within the Public Domain.

*This edition is reprinted for entertainment purposes
and in accordance with all applicable Federal and International Laws.*

Introduction Copyright 2018 by Dahlia V. Nightly

CREDITS & ACKNOWLEDGEMENTS

Front Cover -
Apothecary Card (1864)
From the archives of the *Library of Congress*
[Public Domain]
via Wikimedia Commons

Back Cover -
Imaginary Portrait of Hippocrates
Wellcome Images Iconographic Collections
www.WellcomeImages.org
[CC BY 4.0 - https://creativecommons.org/licenses/by/4.0],
via Wikimedia Commons

Black Books Logo -
Candle Collection by VectorPocket, via FreePik.com (Cropped)

Marbled Pedestal with Old Books by Kues1, via FreePik.com (Cropped)

Vanitas [Painting] by Bartholomäus Bruyn the Elder,
[Public Domain] via Wikimedia Commons (Cropped)

Research / Sources -
Wikimedia Commons
www.Commons.Wikimedia.org

Many thanks to all the incredible photographers, artists,
researchers, and archivists who share their great work.

PLEASE NOTE :
As with all reprinted books of this age that are intended to perfectly reproduce the original edition, considerable pains and effort had to be undertaken to correct fading and sometimes outright damage to existing proofs of this title. At times, this task can be quite monumental, requiring an almost total rebuilding of some pages from digital proofs of multiple copies. Despite this, imperfections still sometimes exist in the final proof and may detract slightly from the visual appearance of the text.

DISCLAIMER :
Due to the age of this book, some methods or practices may have been deemed unsafe or unacceptable in the interim years. In utilizing the information herein, you do so at your own risk. We republish antiquarian books without judgment or revisionism, solely for their historical and cultural importance, and for educational purposes.

Strange Arts for Dark Hearts

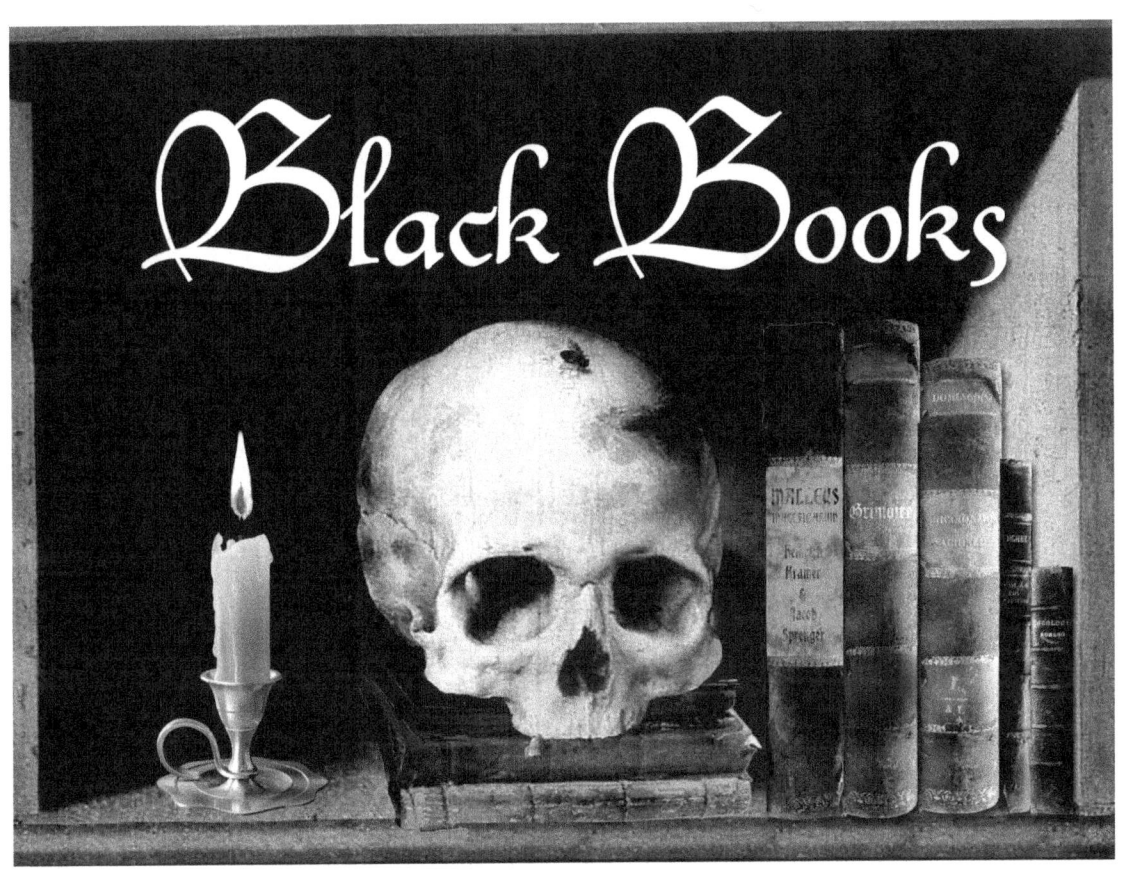

Black Books
PUBLICATIONS

Introduction

We at *Black Books* are pleased to bring you this special edition of fantastic a old book on the history of medicine and the superstitions surrounding it.

This special edition of **Superstitions Connected with the History and Practice of Medicine and Surgery** was written by Thomas Joseph Pettigrew, and first published in 1844, making it over 170 years old.

This fascinating antiquarian text covers topics like *Origin of Chemistry, Alchemy of Egyptian Origin, Sol-Lunar Influence Upon Diseases, Holy Cures, Hippocrates the First Physician to Relieve Medicine from the Trammels of Superstition, Magic and Divination, Talismans, Amulets, Charms, Of the Influence of the Mind Upon the Body*, and many more.

This old book smashes the genre-boundary and will appeal to so many different people with different areas of interest like the history of medicine, alchemy, magic, divination, surgery, psychology, astrology, and superstitions, among other subjects. This is an absolute essential read for all those enthusiastic about the history of both medicine and superstitions.

Strangely yours...

~ Dahlia V. Nightly

State of Jefferson, August 2018

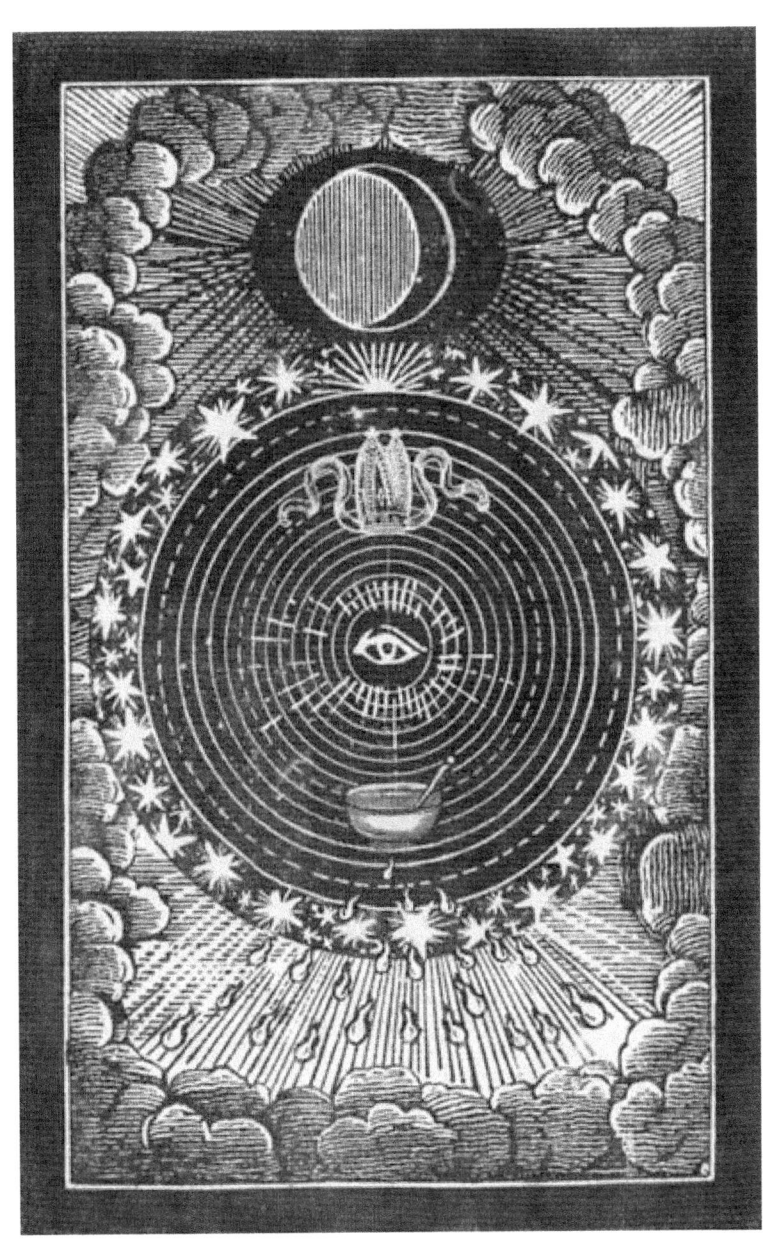

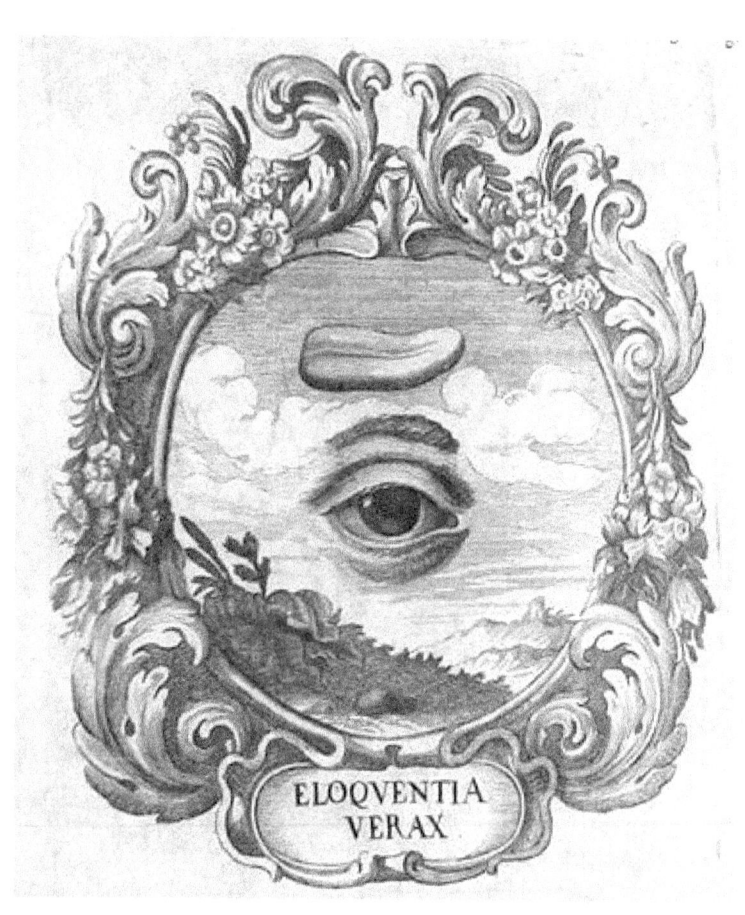

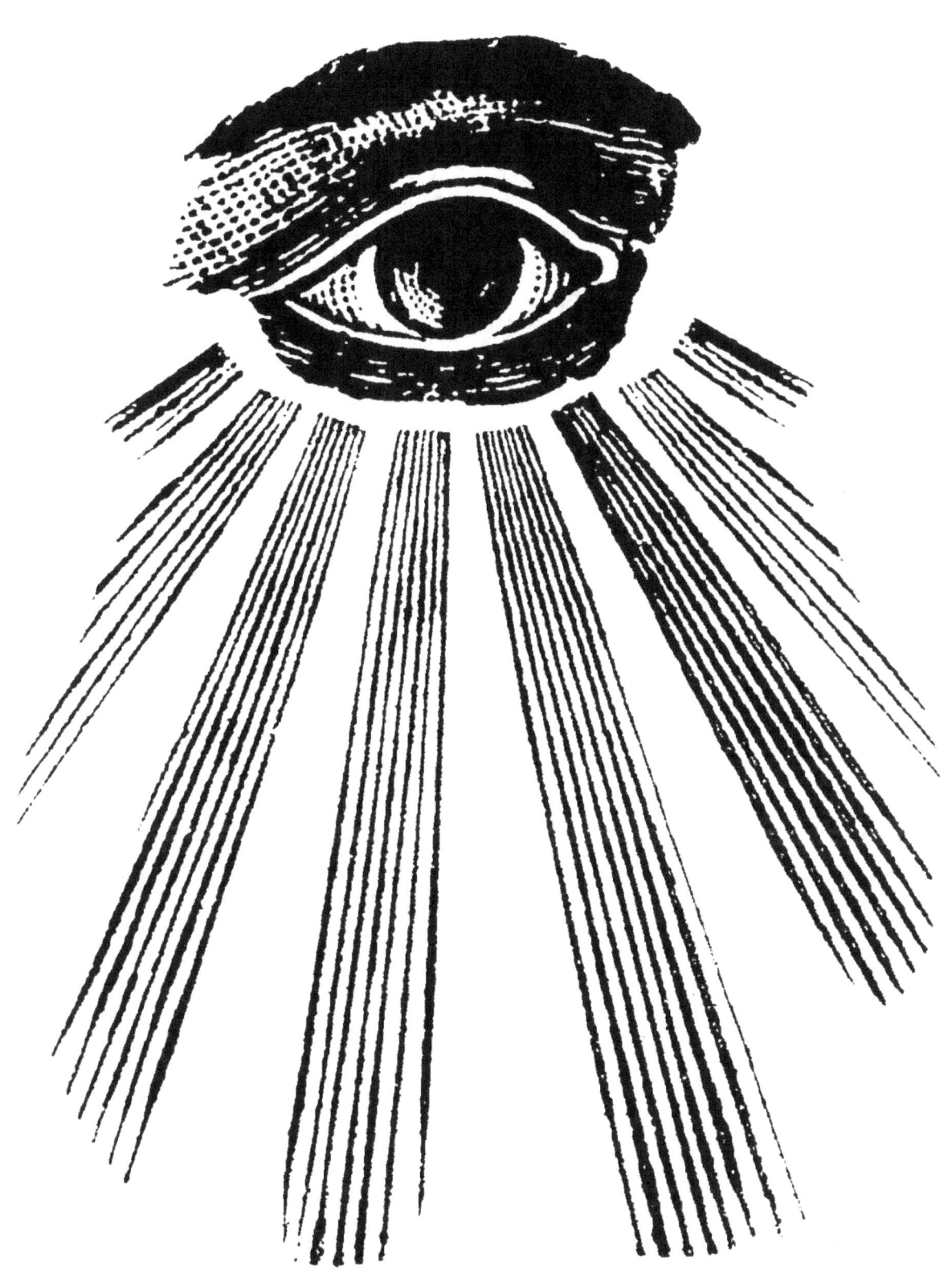

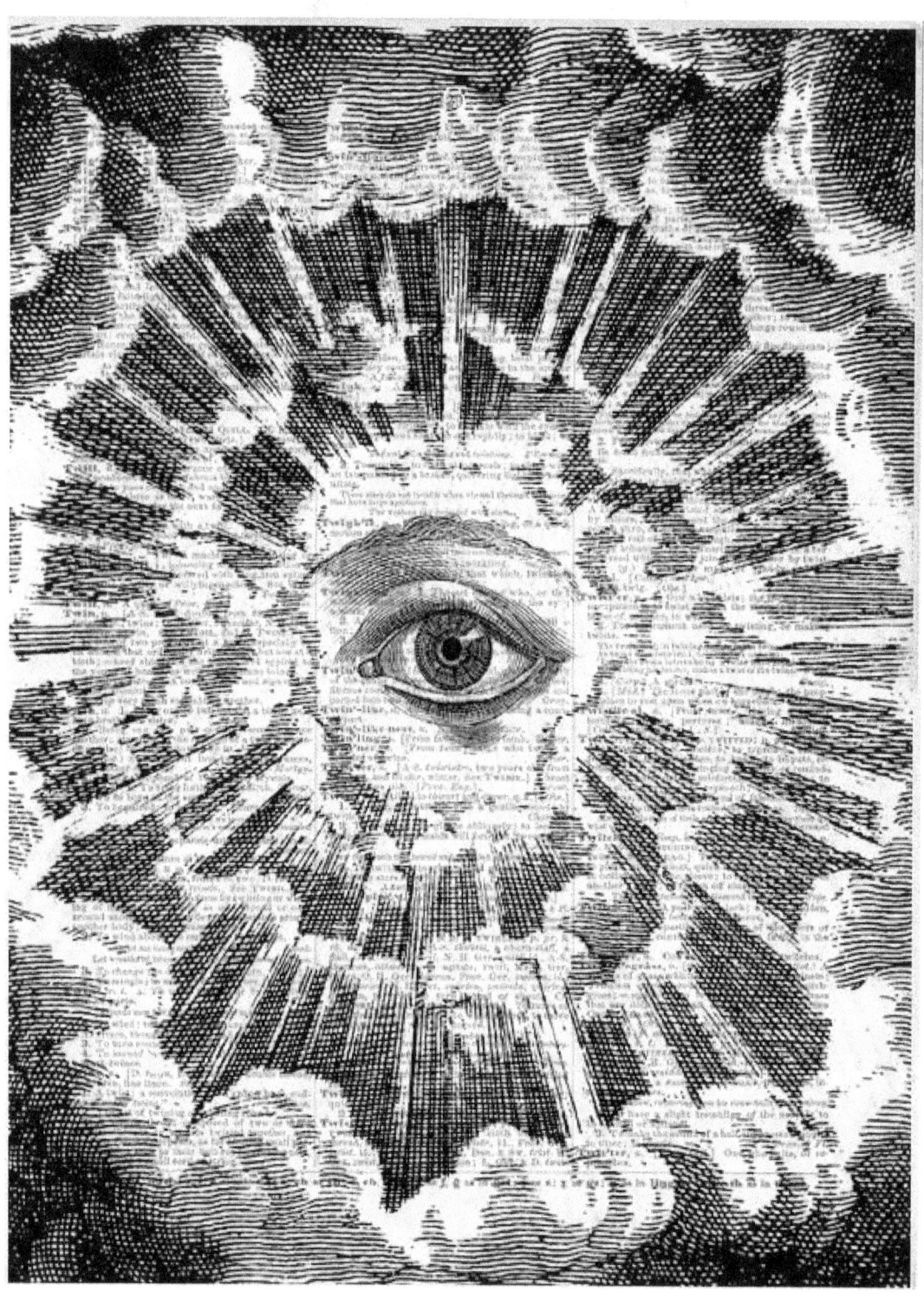

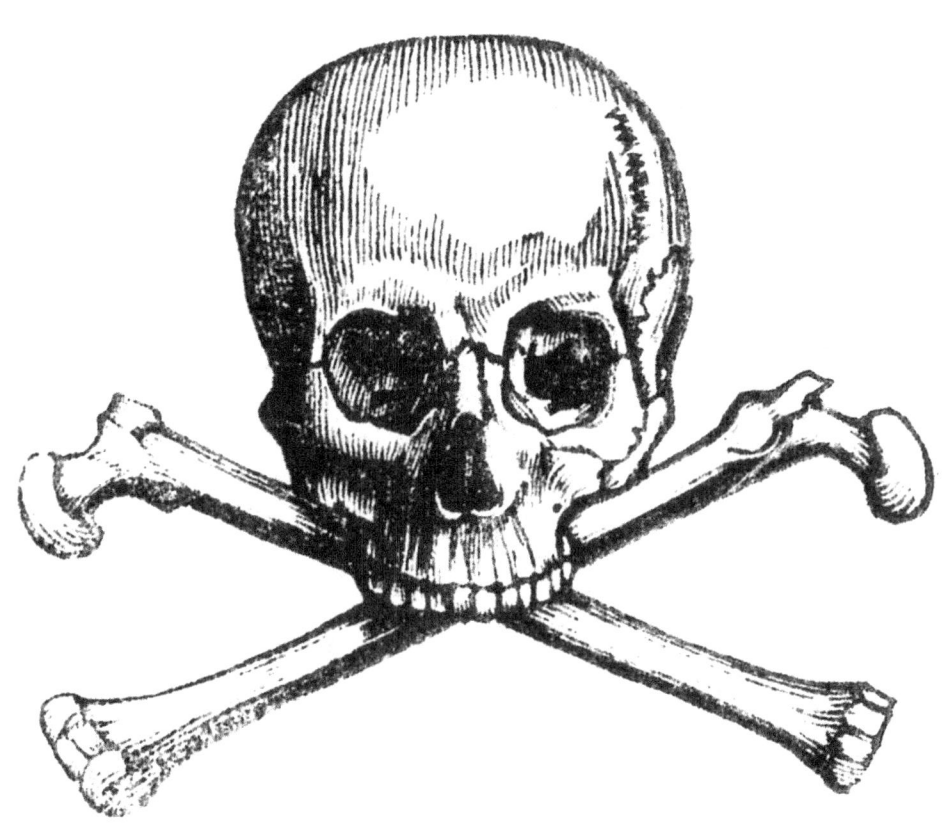

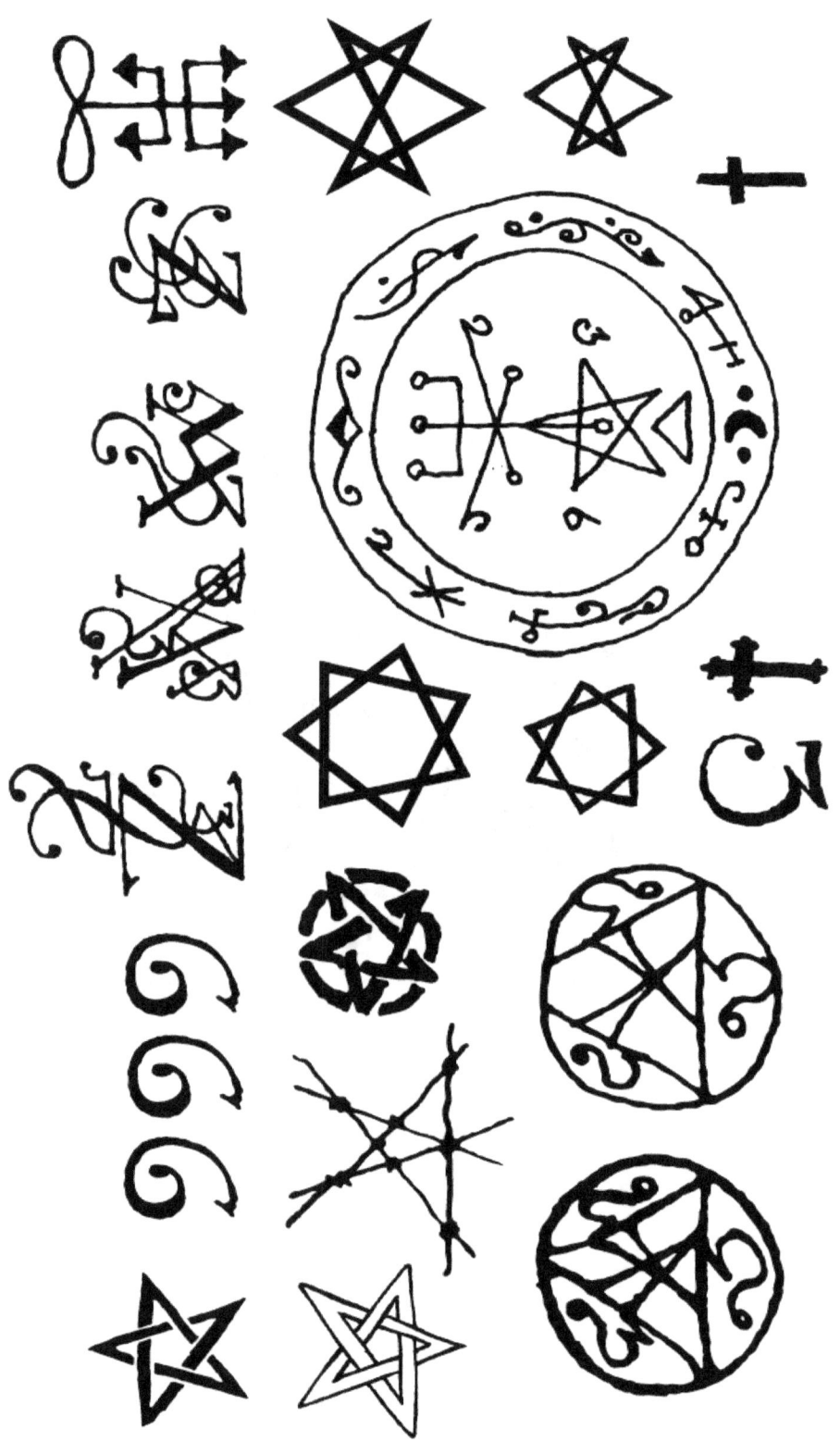

DEDICATION.

TO

HUDSON GURNEY, ESQ., F.R.S., V.P.S.A.,

ETC., ETC., ETC.

My dear Sir,

I eagerly embrace the opportunity afforded me by the publication of these pages on the Superstitions connected with the History of Medicine and Surgery, to inscribe them to one, whose varied information and powerful intellect qualify him to form so able a judgment on the subject. Had I not, however, equal assurance of the benevolent disposition of your mind as of your ability, I should fear the result of my boldness.

Whatever may be the opinion your knowledge of History and Antiquities may lead you to form of my little production, written amidst the interruptions of a professional life, it is extremely gratifying to me to have the opportunity of publicly recording with what regard and esteem,

I have the honour to be,

Your most faithful and obliged servant,

T. J. PETTIGREW.

Saville Row, Oct. 28, 1843.

CONTENTS.

	PAGE
INTRODUCTION :—Value of Health—Veneration for Physicians—Empiricism—Paracelsus; his character—The 'Six follies of Science'—Speculative Conceits of Learned Men . . .	13–17
ALCHYMY :—Origin of Chemistry—Geber—Alchymy of Egyptian origin; evidence of it afforded by the Enchorial Manuscripts; propagated by the Arabians—Objects of the Alchymists—The most celebrated—Royal Alchymists—Elias Ashmole; his 'Theatrum Chemicum Britannicum'—Philosopher's Stone—Mineral Stone—Vegetable Stone—Magical or Prospective Stone—Angelical Stone—Secresy of the Alchymists—Eminent Men chargeable with the folly—Girtanner's Prophecy . . .	18–31
ASTROLOGY :—Origin of Talismans—Doctrine of Signatures—Planetary Influence—Sol-Lunar Influence upon Diseases—Colours of Substances—Gathering of Plants . . .	32–40

EARLY MEDICINE AND SURGERY :—Ridiculous Speculations—Surgical Instruments—Combined Duties of Physician and Surgeon; when separated—First Surgical Operation—Royal Egyptian Physician wrote on Anatomy—Practice of Medicine with the Priesthood—Supposed Celestial Influence in the production of Diseases—Theological Anatomy—Appropriation of parts of the Body to various Deities—Zodiacal Constellation—Hippocrates the first physician to relieve Medicine from the trammels of superstition—Egyptian Æsculapius—Magic and Di-

CONTENTS.

	PAGE
vination—Prohibition of Priests to practice Medicine and Surgery—Various Decrees of Councils to effect the same—Miraculous Cures by the Interposition of Saints—Particular Saints for special diseases—Holy Cures—Holy Wells and Fountains—Relics of Saints	41–61
TALISMANS :—Cabalistical Characters—Astronomical—Magical—Mixed—Sigilla Planetarum—Hebrew Names and Characters—Phylacteries—Characts	62–65
AMULETS :—Eastern origin—Various kinds—Grigris—Odd Numbers—Abraxas—Abracadabra	66–76
CHARMS :—Origin of the term—Charm for Luxation ; for Protection against Diseases in general ; against Accidents ; against Malignant Influences—Evil Eye—Epilepsy—Convulsions and Fits—Hysteria—St. Vitus's Dance—Madness—Palsy— Sciatica—Lameness—Headach—Toothach — Plague—Fevers—Ague—Hectic Fever and Consumption—Glacach—Hooping-cough — Gout —Scrofula—Rickets—Sore Eyes—Marasmus—Calculus—Cholera—Jaundice—Worms—Venomous Bites—Tarantula—Erysipelas—Burns—Thorns —Warts—Smallpox—Hemorrhage and Hemorrhoids—Sterility—Childbirth—Child's Caul—Cramp—Incubus	77–118
ON THE INFLUENCE OF THE MIND UPON THE BODY :—Power of the Imagination—Effects of Terror upon the Colour of the Hair ; in dissipating Pain ; in curing Diseases—Anger—Grief—Fear — Joy — Sudden Death—Sympathies—Passions productive of Diseases—Effects of Imagination — Metallic Tractors — Medical Faith—Religious Feeling—Prince Hohenlohe's Cases—Importance of attending to the mental Condition of the Sick	119–152
ROYAL GIFT OF HEALING :—A practice of English growth—commenced with Edward the Confessor and continued to the time of Queen Anne—French kings practised it—Historical evidences—Error of Dr. Plot—Presentation of a	

CONTENTS.

PAGE

Piece of Gold—Origin of English Gold Coinage—Touch-pieces of Charles II, James II, Anne, and the Pretender—Medical Authorities: Gilbertus Anglicus; John of Gaddesden—Clerical and Legal Authorities; Peter de Blois; Archbishop Bradwardine; Sir John Fortescue—Henry VII establishes a particular ceremony at the Healings—its variations in the time of Charles II and Queen Anne—Proclamations preserved in the State Paper Office relating to the Cure of the King's Evil—most extensively practised by Charles II—Browne's Adenochoiradelogia—Trial of Thomas Rosewell for denying the power of Charles to heal—practised by the Pretenders—Carte deprived of the subscription of the City of London to his History, for giving countenance to the power of the Stuarts—Cessation of the practice upon the accession of the House of Brunswick . . 153-198

VALENTINE GREATRAKES' CURES:—His character—Attestations to his practice—John Leverett's Manual Exercise 199-200

SYMPATHETICAL CURES:—Sir Kenelm Digby; his Discourse at Montpellier—Mr. Howell's case—Attempted explanation—The doctrine of ancient origin—Weapon Salve; Dryden's notice of it in the 'Tempest'—Real explanation of Sympathetical Cures—Advancement of Surgery—Doctrine of Adhesion—Restoration of parts—Remarkable instances of the Union of severed parts, the Nose, the Ear, Fingers, &c. 201-213

SUPERSTITIONS

CONNECTED WITH

MEDICINE AND SURGERY.

INTRODUCTION.

"Man is a dupeable animal. Quacks in medicine, quacks in religion, and quacks in politics know this, and act upon that knowledge. There is scarcely any one who may not, like a trout, be taken by tickling."

SOUTHEY.

WHEN we consider that health has ever been looked upon as the first of all blessings, we cannot be surprised at the regard, esteem, and even veneration which have been paid to those who have successfully devoted themselves to the removal or relief of disease. "Homines ad Deos nullâ re proprius accedunt, quam salutem hominibus dando,"* is the expressed opinion of the

---

* [Men resemble the Gods in nothing so much as in giving health to their fellow men.]

celebrated Roman orator. Medicine, however, has been, and still continues to be, an art so conjectural and uncertain, that our astonishment at the anxiety with which empirics have been sought after and followed is much diminished. Regular professional men are too sensible of the deficiencies, and too keenly alive to the uncertainty of the power of medicines over disease, to venture to speak boldly and decisively so as to gain the entire confidence of their patients, whose natural irritability is perhaps, under the influence of disease, much excited, increased, and aggravated. The bold and unblushing assertion of the empiric of a neverfailing remedy,* constantly reiterated, inspires confidence in the invalid, and not unfrequently tends by its operation on the mind to assist in the eradication of disorder. Few people possess either leisure or inclination in large and populous places, where alone the quack sets upon his work of deception and not unfrequently destruction, to examine into and detect the imposition. Human credulity is too strong to resist the bold and unblushing assertions of the empiric, and to his hands is readily committed the care of the most precious gift of Heaven.

It has not inaptly been observed,† that "in the true infancy of science, philosophers were

---

* Death is the cure of all diseases. There is no *catholicon* or universal remedy I know, but this, which though nauseous to queasy stomachs, yet to prepared appetites is nectar, and a pleasant potion of immortality." (Browne's Religio Medici.)

† D'Israeli's Curiosities of Literature, second series, vol. iii., p. 1.

as imaginative a race as poets." No discovery, in short, was promulgated but in combination with the marvellous. Hence the 'Admirable Secrets' of Albertus Magnus; the 'Natural Magic' of Baptista Porta; the 'Demones of Cornelius Agrippa; the 'Elixir of Life' of Van Helmont; and the 'Fairy' of Paracelsus. It would be no easy task to assign the earliest age of quackery in medicine. It is, perhaps, coeval with the introduction of chemistry, but the first renowned quack is probably to be found in Paracelsus. He boasted his power of making man immortal, yet he died at the early age of 48 years, in the hospital of St. Sebastian, at Saltzburg in Germany, in the year 1541, having followed a life of great indulgence and dissipation. It is not a little singular that the family name of this "strange and paradoxical genius" should have been *Bombastus*, which he changed, as was a common practice of the times in which he lived, to another, and assumed that of Paracelsus. His zeal and application were extraordinary. He derived his knowledge from travelling in various parts of the world, and consulting monks, conjurors, barber-surgeons, old women, and all persons said to be gifted with the knowledge of secret arts, remedies, &c. He was professor of medicine at Basle, but became renowned by a nostrum called *azoth*, which he vaunted as the philosopher's stone — the medical panacea — the tincture of life. He styled himself the "monarch of physicians," and arrogantly exclaimed that the hair on the back of his head knew more than all authors;

that the clasps of his shoes were more learned than Galen or Avicenna; and that his beard possessed more experience than all the academy of Basle: " Stultissimus pilus occipitis mei plus scit, quam omnes vestri doctores, et calceorum meorum annuli doctiores sunt quam vester Galenus et Avicenna, barba mea plus experta est quam vestræ omnes Academiæ." Extravagant as all this may appear, it yet had the effect of dissipating a too excessive admiration of the ancients, at that time prevalent in the schools. His boldness was such, that at his first lecture upon his appointment to the professorship in the University, he, before his pupils, publicly burnt the writings of Galen and Avicenna! His education, however, was very imperfect, and he was ignorant even of his own vernacular tongue. Thomas Erastus, one of his pupils, wrote a book to detect his impostures. He was nevertheless a man of great ability, and did much towards the advancement of chemical knowledge, particularly in its application to the purposes of medicine. Armed with opium, antimony, and mercury, he effected many extraordinary cures.

The quadrature of the circle; the multiplication of the cube; the perpetual motion; the philosophical stone; magic; and judicial astrology have been aptly denominated "The Six Follies of Science." However vain has been the study, and however futile the results, the indulgence of the vanity and the pains of the research have not been unattended with benefit to mankind; inasmuch as they have been the cause of many discoveries of much importance. The errors in medicine have usually originated in the speculative conceits of men of superior capacities. "The blunders of the weak are short lived, but a false theory, with a semblance of nature, struck in the mint of genius, often deceives the learned, and passes current through the world."

ALCHYMY.

"Trust to this doctrine, set herein your desiers,
And now lerne the regiment of your fiers."
NORTON.

THE study of alchymy gave birth to chemistry; its principal object was the transmutation of the baser metals into gold and silver. Suidas, whose Greek Lexicon was composed in the twelfth century, has defined chemistry "the preparation of silver and gold:" this is a distinct identification of chemistry with alchymy. A better etymology of the word is to be found, perhaps, in the fact that the country of Egypt was called Khame, Chemia, Chamia, or Cham, the meaning of which in hieroglyphics is black, — an allusion, probably, to the dark soil thrown up by the river Nile; and in this country chemistry may be looked upon to have originated. Chemistry now happily constitutes a science of great practical benefit to mankind, embraces objects of vast extent and utility, gives to us an intimate knowledge of the nature of bodies, and no longer tempts either the superstitious or the avaricious to the attainment of improper, unnatural, or inordinate gains. Dr. Thomson[*] is

---

[*] History of Chemistry, p. 14.

disposed to believe that chemistry or alchymy—understanding by these terms the art of making gold and silver—originated with the Arabians after the establishment of the caliphs, and that its application was then first directed to the purposes of medicine. Geber, who lived in the seventh century, he observes, makes no allusion to the transmutation of metals; and he hence concludes that the practice dates its origin posterior to his time. It must, however, be remarked that Geber expressly mentions the philosopher's stone, and professes to give the mode of preparing it, and I know not how to separate this art from that of converting or altering the nature of different substances. Dr. Thomson regards Geber's work as the earliest chemical treatise in existence; and he describes it as written with so much plainness that we can understand the nature of the substances which he employed, the processes which he followed, and the greater number of the products he obtained. The chemical facts observable in his work he thinks entitle him to the appellation of "The father and founder of chemistry." Yet Dr. Johnson regarded his language as so proverbially obscure, that he presumed the word gibberish or geberish to have arisen from the style of his writings. The language of the alchymists was enigmatical and obscure, their science and all its processes were mysterious, and directed to be conducted with great privacy. The metals were personified—gold was the only pure and healthy man, the others were as "lepers" or diseased ones.

Alchymy cannot be regarded as of Arabian origin, however much it may have been cultivated and extended in that country. It flourished at a very early period in Egypt, and the late discoveries in that "land of marvels" have shown an extended acquaintance with various arts and sciences as exercised in the different manufactures, of which representations are to be found in the tombs and excavations of a very early date. Without some knowledge of chemistry the Egyptians could never have excelled, as they have done, in the making of glass, of linen, in dyeing, in the use of mordaunts, &c. Their manufacture of metals, particularly of gold — the whole process of which is represented in the tombs of Beni Hassan and at Thebes — into various ornaments; their gold wire, their gilding, &c., exhibit great ability, and could not have been effected without some knowledge of metallurgy. Their embalmings also display an acquaintance with chemistry. The Egyptian manuscripts hitherto discovered have not afforded any particular light into the extent of their knowledge; but several papyri have been found to contain certain formulæ; and one, a bilingual manuscript (being Enchorial and Greek) was examined by my late friend, Professor Reuvens, the conservator of the Museum of Antiquities at Leyden, and was found to treat of magical operations, and to contain upwards of one hundred chemical and alchymical formulæ.

It has been usual to ascribe the introduction of alchymy to Pythagoras, to Solomon, or rather to Hermes, and it has not unfrequently been called the hermetical science. Gibbon has shown that the Greeks were inattentive either to the use or the abuse of chemistry, and that the immense collection of Pliny contains no instance of, or reference to, the transmutation of metals. He states the persecution of Diocletian to be the first authentic event in the history of alchymy. After the conquest of Egypt by the Arabs it spread over the globe.

The objects of the alchymists were to convert other metals into gold and silver, to remedy all diseases, and to prolong human life to an indefinite period.

> "A perfect medicine for bodies that be sick
> Of all infirmities to be relieved;
> This heleth nature and prolongeth lyfe eke."

To attain such objects it is not surprising there should have been many aspirants; the credulity of man was speedily excited by the benefits held forth, and for a very long time an almost universal belief in the truth of the propositions was entertained.

The most celebrated ancient alchymists were Albertus Magnus, Roger Bacon, Raymund Lully, Arnoldus de Villa Nova, John Isaac Hollandus, Basil Valentine, Paracelsus, and Van Helmont.

The importance of chemical investigations and processes, as applicable to medicine, was first shown by Paracelsus; metals being exposed by him to the action of different acids, various preparations were made, and are employed in medicine with benefit, to the present day. Tinctures, essences, and extracts have from his time superseded the useless syrups and decoctions previously employed.

The desire of transmuting base metals into gold has called into exercise the worst passions of mankind —

> "To seech by *alkimy* greate ryches to winn."
> (Norton's *Ordinall*, p. 6.)

Thus a love of riches sprang out of the pursuit of chemical science; and, considering the extraordinary operations connected with the study and the decompositions that have been effected, it is perhaps scarcely surprising that so many men of considerable talent should have become so infatuated. Many, doubtless, like Peter Hopkins,[*] studied alchymy for the pure love of speculation and curious inquiry, not with the slightest intention of ever pursuing it for the desire of riches. Many liked it because it was mysterious. There have also been royal alchymists, driven probably to the entertainment of a vain hope by the extravagancies and profligacy of their lives. Henry VI., according to Evelyn,[†] endeavoured to recruit his empty coffers by recourse to alchymy. Henry IV., had enacted a statute prohibiting the craft of multiplication. None were permitted to multiply gold or silver under pain of felony. Henry VI. repealed this

---

[*] Doctor, vol. iii., p. 102.

[†] Numismata. Also, D'Israeli, Curios. of Lit., vol. i., p. 498.

statute and published a patent *authoritate Parliamenti*, which has been given by Prynne in his 'Aurum Reginæ,' and in which the monarch tells his subjects that the happy hour was drawing nigh, when, by the discovery of the philosopher's stone, he should be enabled to pay all the debts of the nation in real gold and silver.

Elias Ashmole, who styles himself Mercuriophilus Anglicus, has collected together in his 'Theatrum Chemicum Britannicum' (Lond. 1652, 4to.), many curious poetical* pieces on alchymy. He states that his adopted father, Backhouse, an astrologer, bequeathed to him, *in syllables*, the true matter of the philosopher's stone as a legacy; by which, as D'Israeli says, "we learn that a miserable wretch knew the art of making gold, yet always lived a beggar; and that Ashmole really imagined he was in possession of the syllables of a secret;" thus verifying Ben Jonson's lines addressed to the alchymists.

"If all you boast of your great art be true,
Sure, willing poverty lives most in you."

The work of Ashmole to which I have alluded is perhaps the most curious record we have of the history of the follies, vain conceits, and incredible belief of the alchymists. He speaks with great caution of the philosopher's stone,

* His reason for selecting poetical pieces is thus given: "To prefer prose before poetry is no other or better than to let a rough-hewen clowne take the wall of a rich-clad lady of honour, or to hang a presence chamber with tarpalin instead of tapestry."

"knowing enough to hold his tongue, but not enough to speake." Of its powers, however, he gives a particular account — as, he says, "a philosophical account of that eminent secret treasured up in the bosome of nature, which hath been sought for of many, but found by few." He describes also the mineral stone, the vegetable stone, the magical stone, and the angelicall stone; and prior to his description he solemnly tells us, "Incredulity is given to the world as a punishment."

The *mineral stone* hath the power of transmuting any imperfect earthy matter into its utmost degree of perfection; that is, to convert the basest of metals into perfect gold* and silver; flints into all manner of precious stones, as rubies, sapphires, emeralds, diamonds, &c.

The *vegetable stone*, by which Abraham, Moses, and Solomon wrought many wonders. The nature of man, beasts, fowls, fishes, all kinds of trees, plants, flowers, &c., may by this stone be made to grow, flourish, and bear fruit, — increase in colour, smell, &c., when and where and at whatever season of the year its possessor may please.

The *magical or perspective stone* makes a strict inquisition, discovers any person in any part of the world whatever, and enables you to understand the language of birds, beasts, &c.

The *angelicall stone* can neither be felt, seen, or weighed, but it can be tasted. It will lodge

---

* "Gold, I confesse, is a delicious object, a goodly light, which we admire and gaze upon *ut pueri in Junonis avem*."

in the fire to eternity without being prejudiced. It hath a divine power, celestial and invisible, and endows the possessor with divine gifts. It affords the apparition of angels, and gives a power of conversing with them by dreams and revelations, nor dare any evil spirit approach the place where it is.

In addition to the stones already noticed, particular mention is made by various professors of alchymy of *white* and *red* stones: thus —

> "Thei said that within the center of incomplete white
> Was hid our *red stone* of most delight;
> Which maie, with strength and kinde of fier,
> Be made to appeare right as we desier.
> *Pandulphus* in *turba* saide, *mente secura,*
> *Et ejus umbra in vera tinctura.*
> *Maria* confirmed it *in fide ocultata,*
> *Quod in ipsa albedine est rubedo ocultata.*
> The boke *Laudabile Sanctum*, made by *Hermes,*
> Of the *Red Worke*, speaketh in this wise:
> *Candida tunc rubeo jacet uxor nupta marito,*
> That is to saie, if ye take heede thereto,
> Then is the faire white woman
> Married to the ruddy man.
> Understandinge thereof if ye would gett,
> When our *white stone* shall suffer heate,
> And rest in fier as red as blood,
> Then is the marriage perfect and good;
> And ye maie trewly know that tyme
> How the seminall seed masculine
> Hath wrought and won the victory
> Upon the menstrualls worthily,
> And well converted them to his kinde,
> As by experience ye shall finde,
> Passing the substance of the *embrion,*
> For then compleate is made our stone;
> Whom wise men said that ye shoulde feede
> With his own venome when it is neede.

> Then ride or go where ye delight,
> For all your costs he woll you quite.
> Thus endeth the subtill worke with all her store,
> I need not, I maie not, I woll show no more."
>
> (Norton's *Ordinall*, p. 90.)

Ashmole makes an apology for the quaintness of the style of his work. "The style and language thereof," says he, "may, I confesse, to some seem irkesome and uncouth, and so it is indeed to those that are strangers thereunto, but withal very significant. *Old* words have a strong *emphasis;* others may look upon them as rubbish or trifles, but they are grossly mistaken; for what some light braines may esteem as foolish toyes, deeper judgments can and will value as sound and serious matter."

Alchymists were advised to be particularly select in the choice of their assistants. Norton says —

> "Noe minister is apt to this intent,
> But he be sober, wise, and diligent;
> Trewe and watchfull and also timerous,
> Close of tongue, of body not vitious,
> Clenely of hands in tuching curious,
> Not disobedient, neither presumptuous."
>
> (*Ordinall*, p. 93.)

An anonymous alchymist, the writer of the *Pater Sapientiæ,* repeatedly recommends secrecy to the adepts:

> "Be thou in a place secret, by thyselfe alone,
> That noe man see or hear what thow schalt say or done.'

> "Trust not thy friend too much, wheresoere thow goe,
> For he that thow trustest best, sometyme may be thy foe."
>
> (p. 194.)

"Therefore kepe close of thy tongue and of thy hand,
From the officers and governours of the land;
And from other men, that they of thy craft nothing know,
For in wytnes thereof they wyll thee hang and draw."

(p. 196.)

"Therefore make no man of the councell rude nor rustie,
But him that thow knowest both true and trustie;
In ryding and going, sleeping and waking,
Both in worde and deede and in hys disposing.

"Also in thy own chamber looke thow be secret,
That thy dores and windowes be close shut;
For some wyll come and look in every corner,
And anon they will aske what thow makest there."

(p. 208.)

Chaucer, who is said to have studied alchymy under Gower, expresses the same in a better manner:

"Make privy to your dealing as few as you maie,
For three may keepe councell if twain be awaie."

Sir Thomas Browne gave much assistance to his friends engaged in the pursuit of alchymy, and it is scarcely possible to suppose him not to have been tinctured in some degree with the prevailing opinions of his age. He was intimate with Dr. Arthur Dee, son of the celebrated Dr. John Dee, who held a firm belief as to the transmutation of base metals into gold and silver, which he declared to Sir Thomas he had "ocularly, undeceivably, and frequently beheld."*

* Suppl. Mem. by Mr. Wilkin, p. xcv.

The vagaries of the philosophers in search of the wonderful stone, to us of the present day appears an extraordinary and almost inconceivable delusion. That men of enlightened minds, and extensive and profound learning, should have pursued an object so visionary, tends only to excite in us a feeling bordering on contempt; yet has science derived real and substantial advantages from their anile conceits, and important discoveries have emanated from their fruitless attempts.

A belief in the philosopher's stone lasted for a very long period, and the memory of several eminent men is chargeable with the folly. Lord Bacon speculated upon it, and Sir Isaac Newton is said once to have entertained the possibility of finding it, and that he also acknowledged that the idle and vain pursuit of astrology had led him to cultivate astronomy. "The sons of chymistry," says Lord Bacon,* "while they are busy seeking the hidden gold, whether real or not, have, by turning over and trying, brought much profit and convenience to mankind."

With such fruits as the result, let us be charitable to those who first promulgated the desire; examining, as we ought to do, in the most scrupulous manner, every subject connected with credulity and superstition, and separating the endeavours of the enthusiastic philosophers to extend the sphere of human knowledge, from the mercenary attempts of inter-

---

* Interpretation of Nature.

ested and unprincipled hypocrites, ever alive and ready to prey upon the weakness of human nature.

Arnoldus de Villa Nova, a celebrated physician, who lived in the thirteenth and fourteenth centuries, and well known by his 'Commentary on the School of Salernum,' was the teacher of Raymund Lully, and highly renowned in his day as an alchymist and astrologer. He entertained the vain idea of having discovered the secret of the transmutation of metals into gold, and he confidently predicted by his astrological acumen the destruction of the world in the year 1335. His alchymical speculations were productive of many advantages, and chemistry is indebted to him for the discovery of the sulphuric, the muriatic, and the nitric acids. The sulphuric acid he found to be a menstruum capable of retaining the sapid and odoriferous principles of various vegetable substances, and from this discovery have issued the numerous spirituous solutions so commonly used as tinctures in medicine, and as cosmetics. The essential oil of turpentine was also discovered by him, and he is said to have been the first to give any regular scientific details of the process of distillation. This case is one, out of many others that might be referred to, illustrative of the advantages science has received through the ridiculous expectations of the alchymists.

The nineteenth century has not yet passed away, and Dr. Christopher Girtanner, an eminent professor of Gottingen, has prophesied, in a Memoir on Azote, in the 'Annales de Chimie,'

No. 100, that it will give birth to the transmutation of metals. The passage expressing this extraordinary opinion is too singular not to be here transcribed:

"In the nineteenth century the transmutation of metals will be generally known and practised. Every chemist and every artist will make gold; kitchen utensils will be of silver, and even gold, which will contribute more than anything else to prolong life, poisoned at present by the oxyds of copper, lead, and iron, which we daily swallow with our food."

It is no part of my intention to compose a history of the alchymists, and I shall therefore quit the subject by enumerating a piece of folly, not to say imposture, recorded of Edward Kelley, the companion of the renowned Dr. Dee. Kelley, willing to make what alchymists call a projection, is said to have cut a piece of metal out of a warming-pan, which, having placed on the fire and endowed it with a small portion of his elixir, was instantly transmuted into a plate of pure silver! This was sent, together with the remains of the warming-pan, to Queen Elizabeth, as a successful exercise of his power. He professed equal ability in the formation of gold, and gave away upon occasion of the marriage* of one of his maid servants, rings, twisted with three gold wires, to the value of £4000, which, as Ashmole observes, "was highly generous, but

* This was at Trebona, in 1589.

to say truth, openly profuse beyond the modest limits of a sober philosopher."*

* Eusèbe Salverte published, in 1829, at Paris, a work entitled 'Des Sciences Occultes, ou Essai sur la Magie, les Prodiges, et les Miracles,' which will reward the reader's patient attention. He will there find an immense collection of curious subjects discussed with considerable ability, and he will be enabled to appreciate the extent of knowledge possessed by the ancients in different branches of natural philosophy — mechanics, acoustics, optics, hydrostatics, chemistry, medicine, and meteorology.

ASTROLOGY.

"If either Sextus Empiricus, Picus Mirandula, Sextus ab Heminga, Pererius, Erastus, Chambers, &c., have so far prevailed with any man that he will attribute no virtue at all to the Heavens, or to Sun, or Moon, more than he doth to their signs at an innkeeper's post, or tradesman's shop, or generally condemn all such astrological aphorisms approved by experience; I refer him to Bellantius, Pirovanus, Marascallerus, Goclenius, Sir Christopher Heydon, &c."

BURTON'S ANATOMY OF MELANCHOLY.

ALCHYMY, judicial astrology, and natural magic are all intimately associated together. "Judiciall astrologie," according to Ashmole, "is the key of naturall magick, and naturall magick the doore that leads to this blessed (the philosopher's) stone." In the employment of certain characters, letters, words, or figures, as talismans, to avert or conquer disease, it is pretended that they have been derived from the various appearances to be observed upon certain plants, roots, seeds, fruits, &c., even upon stones, flints, and other bodies. These figures, the astrologers contend, are the evidence of Providence, and not the result of chance, and directed to our good, being the characters and figures of those stars by whom they are principally governed and endowed with particular virtues. "The soule of the world," says Ashmole, "is not confined, nor the celestial influences limited, but can communicate their virtues alike to things *artificially* made as well as *naturally* generated;" from which it is deduced as necessary, that a "fit election" must be built up from the foundation of astrology suitable to the nature of the operation proposed to be effected, and that the stars finding a figure aptly disposed for receiving them, they forthwith impress their virtue, which they retaining, do afterwards operate in that which they find to be "semblable."

Talismans, or the doctrine of signatures, may therefore be said to have taken their origin from a belief that medicinal substances bore upon their external surfaces the properties or virtues they possessed, impressed upon them by planetary influence. The connexion of the properties of substances with their colour is also an opinion of great antiquity: white was regarded as refrigerant, red as hot — hence cold and hot qualities were attributed to different medicines. This opinion led to serious errors in practice. Red flowers were given for disorders of the sanguiferous system, yellow ones for those of the biliary secretion, &c. We find that in small-pox red bed-coverings were employed, with the view of bringing the pustules to the surface of the body. The bed-furniture and hangings were very commonly of a red colour, — red substances were to be looked upon by the patient. Burnt purple, pomegranate seeds, mulberries, or other red ingredients were dissolved in their drink. In short, as Avicenna contended that red bodies moved the blood, everything of a red colour was employed in these cases. John of Gaddesden, physician to Edward II., directs his patients to be wrapped up in scarlet dresses; and he says, that "when the son of the renowned king of England (Edw. II.) lay sick of the small-pox I took care that everything around the bed should be of a red colour; which succeeded so completely that the Prince was restored to perfect health, without a vestige of a pustule remaining." Wraxall, in his 'Memoirs,' says that the Emperor Francis I., when infected with the small-pox, was rolled up in a scarlet cloth, by order of his physician, so late as 1765, when he died. Kæmpfer (History of Japan) says, that "when any of the emperor's children are attacked with the small-pox, not only the chamber and bed are covered with red hangings, but all persons who approach the sick prince must be clad in scarlet gowns." Flannel dyed nine times in blue was held to be efficacious in the removal of glandular swellings.

The rising and setting of the stars, the eclipses of the sun and moon, the appearance of comets or other fiery meteors, the aspects, conjunctions, and oppositions of the planets have all been considered to be intimately influential in the production as in the relief of diseases. Fracastorius, a poet and physician, sought for the causes of diseases in the heavens. Certain positions of the celestial bodies he considered to be of malignant influence, by which contagious disorders were produced. A conjunction of many stars under the large fixed stars predicted a contagion, falling stars and comets denoted putrefaction. The Jesuit Kircher, after a strict examination of almanacs and astrological tables, contended that putrid diseases had always prevailed at those times when the planet Mars and Saturn were in conjunction. He therefore inferred that those two planets emitted very deadly exhalations, which infected the air and all terrestrial productions with a putrescent tendency, — when myriads of animalcules were instantly generated, and the plague, the small-pox, the measles, or some other putrid fevers became inevitable.

Mr. Fraser* notices the superstitious belief of the natives of Khorasan in the powers of the celestial bodies, and says they attributed the ravages of the cholera with which they were visited to the influence of the star Canopus, (called by the Persians and Arabians Zoheil,) which became visible at this time above the horizon, a little before sunrise. The Druids are known to have introduced many superstitions in connexion with the moon, some of which have descended to the present day. Animals were killed, seeds were sown, plants were gathered, timber was felled, voyages were undertaken, new garments were put on, the hair was cut, only at particular periods of the moon. The early English almanacs abound with reference to its condition. Brandt† quotes from 'The Husbandman's Practice, or Prognostication for ever' (Lond. 1664, 8vo.), the following curious passage: " Good to purge with electuaries, the moon in Cancer; with pills, the moon

* Narrative of a Journey into Khorasān, p. 64.
† Popular Antiquities, vol. ii., p. 470.

in Pisces; with potions, the moon in Virgo; good to take vomits, the moon being in Taurus, Virgo, or the latter part of Sagittarius; to purge the head by sneezing, the moon being in Cancer, Leo, or Virgo; to stop fluxes and rheumes, the moon being in Taurus, Virgo, or Capricorne; to bathe when the moon is in Cancer, Libra, Aquarius, or Pisces; to cut the hair off the head or beard when the moon is in Libra, Sagittarius, Aquarius, or Pisces. Briefe observations in husbandry: set, sow seeds, graft, and plant, the moon being in Taurus, Virgo, or in Capricorne; and all kinde of corne, in Cancer; graft in March at the moone's increase, she being in Taurus or Capricorne."

Burton* tells us that St. John's wort, gathered on a Friday, in the horn of Jupiter, when it comes to his effectual operation, (that is, about the full moon in July,) so gathered and borne or hung about the neck, will mightily help melancholy and drive away fantastical spirits.

The influence of the moon in various diseases, particularly those of a pestilential character, has been much remarked by medical practitioners in tropical regions. Dr. Balfour, who for a long time resided at Calcutta, an accurate and intelligent observer of the diseases which occur in hot climates, is generally considered to have satisfactorily established the influence of the moon in cases of fever, and he was induced, during a practice of fourteen years in the East, to pay particular attention to its revolutions in the treatment of these diseases. He found the

* Anatomy of Melancholy, p. 245.

accession of fever to take place during the three days which either precede or follow the full moon; and he has endeavoured to show that at the time of the equinoxes, an additional power is added to the lunar influence exercised on the human frame. These opinions have met with support and received confirmation from the practice and researches of Lind in Bengal, of Cleghorn in Minorca, of Fontana in Italy, of Jackson in Jamaica, of Gillespie at St. Lucia, of Bell in Persia, and of Annesley in Madras. Dr. Moseley carried his opinions with respect to the influence of the moon on mankind to a ridiculous extreme, and affirmed that almost all people of extreme age died at the new or at the full moon. Aristotle ascribes many of the derangements of females to the decrease of the moon. Galen says all animals born when the moon is falciform are weak and feeble, and short lived; whilst those born at the full are the contrary. Lord Bacon invariably fell into a syncope during a lunar eclipse. Vegetable substances, as well as animals, have always been considered to be greatly under the influence of the moon.

It was formerly deemed essential in the cure of diseases to be acquainted with astronomy; and Sir George Ripley, in his 'Compound of Alchimie,' tells us that—

> "A good phisytian who so intendeth to be,
> Our lower astronomy him nedeth well to knowe;
> And after that to lerne, well, urine in a glasse to see,
> And if it neede to be chafed the fyre to blowe,
> Then wyttily it, by divers wayes to throwe,

4

> And after the cause to make a medicine blive,
> Truly telling the ynfirmities all on a rowe:
> Who thus can doe by his physicke is like to thrive."
>
> (p. 114.)

Ashmole declares physic to be "a divine science, even God's theologie; for the Almighty wrote his Scripture in that language before he made Adam to reade it. The ten fathers before the flood, and those that followed, together with Moses and Solomon, were the great physitians in former ages, who bequeathed their heavenly knowledges of naturall helpes to those they judged as well worthy in honesty and industry, as capable thereof: and from their piercing beames all nations enlightened their tapers. Abraham brought it out of Chaldea and bestowed much thereof upon Egypt, and thence a refulgent beame glanced into Greece."*

Hippocrates and Galen held a knowledge of astronomy to be essential to physicians. The latter declares all who are ignorant of it to be no better than homicides: "Homicidas Medicos Astrologiæ ignaros,"† &c. By astronomy these ancient physicians meant astrology. Chaucer, in his picture of a good Physician, says,—

> "With us there was a doctor of phisike;
> In al the world, was thar non hym lyk
> To speke of physik and of surgerye,
> For he wos groundit in astronomie.
> He kept his pacient a ful gret del
> In hourys by his magyk naturel;
> Wel couth he fortunen the ascendent
> Of his ymagys for his pacient."

---

* Page 459.
† De Ingenio Sanitatis, lib. viii., c. 20.

Fabian Withers, speaking of physicians, declares: "So far are they distant from the true knowledge of physic which are ignorant of astrology, that they ought not rightly to be called physicians, but deceivers: for it hath," says he, "been many times experimented and proved that that which many physicians could not cure or remedy with their greatest and strongest medicines, the astronomer hath brought to pass with one simple herb, by observing the moving of the signs." The virtues of herbs were considered to be according to the influence of the planet under which they were sown or gathered. Black hellebore was to be plucked, not cut, and this with the right hand, which was then to be covered with a portion of the robe, and secretly conveyed to the left hand. The person gathering it was also to be clad in white, to be barefooted, and to offer a sacrifice of bread and wine.* Verbena or vervain was to be gathered at the rising of the dog-star, when neither sun nor moon shone, an expiatory sacrifice of fruit and honey having been previously offered to the earth. Hence arose its power to render the possessor invulnerable, to cure fevers, to eradicate poison, and to conciliate friendship. The mistletoe was to be cut with a golden knife, and when the moon should be only six days old.

Uncommon events in barbarous ages were attributed to supernatural agency: hence have arisen the connexion of the names of gods and goddesses with various productions of the earth

---

* Plinii Hist. Nat., lib. xxiv., c. 11.

which have been employed as medicinal agents. The ivy was sacred to Osiris and to Bacchus, the pine to Neptune, the herb mercury to Hermes, black hellebore to Melampus, centuary to Chiron, the laurel to Alorus, the artemesia to Diana, the millefolium to Achilles, the hyacinth to Ajax, the squill to Epimenes, &c. Diseases having been referred to the exercise of supernatural influence, a variety of mysterious rites would be performed to remove them. Superstition is the natural offspring of fear. In savage nations the physicians, if they may be so called, are all conjurors and wizards, persons supposed to be gifted either with divine or demoniacal natures. Incantations, sorcery, jugglery of all kinds, engrafted, probably, in many cases upon enthusiasm, together with ignorance, supply the place of science, to which they are utter strangers. Whatever is beyond their sagacity is assigned to invisible agency. Pliny[*] calls magic the offspring of medicine, and says that after having fortified itself with the help of astrology, it borrowed all its splendour and authority from religion.

[*] Lib. xxix., cap. 1 ; lib. xxx., c. 2.

EARLY MEDICINE AND SURGERY.

"Witches and impostors have always held a competition with physicians."

BACON.

LE CLERC, a physician of considerable eminence and much learning, in his 'Histoire de Médecine,' expressly devotes a chapter to the inquiry,—whether medicine came immediately from God, and how the first remedies were discovered? The first part of the question he determines in the affirmative, and the second he ascribes to the exercise of reason and to chance. Midwifery is generally regarded as a division or department of surgery, manual aid being requisite; and Schultze,* who was professor at the University of Altdorf, has carried his speculations so far back into antiquity as to name Adam the first accoucheur, by the authoritative voice of necessity: " laboranti amicæ obstetricis manus adhibuisse, sicque chirurgiæ primam forte operationem exercuisse." Le Clerc, like a good Frenchman, contends that our first parent was not only the first accoucheur but also the primary physician and surgeon in the world.

* J. H. Schulzii, Historia Medicinæ. Lips. 1728, 4to.; et Italæ, 1742, 8vo.

Surgical instruments are attributed by Brambilla, surgeon to the emperor Francis II. of Austria, to the original invention of Tubal Cain, "the instructor of every artificer in brass and iron." It is singular that among the many implements found in the tombs of Egypt, no instruments that can fairly be denominated surgical have been hitherto discovered; the proficiency of the art of surgery in those early days could not, therefore, have been great. No exemption to the consequences of accidental violence, however, could have been afforded to them, and relief must have been sought for; the causes and effects must have been obvious, and the pain immediate and violent, and would necessarily demand relief. The means employed in the first ages of the world would, we may reasonably infer, be of the most simple kind, and, probably, confined to ablution, suction, and the application of such vegetable productions as were calculated to cool and refresh the injured parts. The offices of the physician and the surgeon were probably combined in the same individual, till a later period, when wars and bloody battles might render the latter a distinct class. The Grecian history affords examples of the practice of the surgeons of early times. In the Iliad, we read that Eurypylus, when wounded with an arrow, thus addressed Patroclus:

> "But thou, Patroclus, act a friendly part,
> Lead to my ships, and draw this deadly dart;
> With lukewarm water wash this gore away,
> With healing balms the raging smart allay,

> Such as sage Chiron, sire of pharmacy,
> Once taught Achilles, and Achilles thee."
>
> (Lib. iv., v., 218.)

When also Menelaus was wounded in the side by an arrow, Machaon, the son of the Grecian Æsculapius, after washing the wound and sucking out the blood, applied a dressing to appease the pain, of the juice of roots bruised, the principal remedy then known:

> "Then suck'd the blood, and sovereign balm infused,
> Which Chiron gave, and Æsculapius used."

Arctinus, a Greek poet, who wrote on the destruction of Troy, is referred to by Dr. W. C. Taylor, in a paper on the ballad literature of Greece;[*] and from the following quotation it would appear that in those early days the medical profession was distinguished from the surgical, and that it was deemed the higher science. Arctinus thus speaks of Podalirius and Machaon:

> "Their father, Neptune, on them both illustrious gifts bestow'd,
> But those of Podalirius the more important show'd.
> Machaon got a skilful hand to heal a wounded part,
> To soothe its pain, and extricate from flesh the barbed dart;
> But Podalirius was taught the secret ills to scan,
> Which work unseen within the frame, and waste the inner man.
> 'Twas he who first the symptoms knew of fatal rage reveal'd
> In Ajax, son of Telamon, lord of the sevenfold shield."

---

[*] Bentley's Miscellany for November, 1842.

Until anatomy was cultivated, surgery could make but little progress, and few operations could be performed. Circumcision is the first surgical operation on record; it was of a simple description, and this, as a holy rite, was executed by the priests. The early constitution of Egypt, as shown by the chronicle of Manetho, who lived 261 A.C. and other existing records, was hierarchical; and a sovereign is mentioned by the chronicler, as having composed some books on anatomy. This sovereign was Athotis, the son of Menes, or, as it is written on the monuments, Menai, the first king of Egypt and the founder of Memphis. Athotis is reported to have been the builder of the palace of Memphis, to have been a physician, and the writer of some anatomical works. He is the same as Thoth I. In later times, according to Herodotus, a particular and minute division of labour characterized the Egyptians; the science of medicine was distributed into different parts; every physician was for one disease — not more; so that every place was full of physicians; for some were doctors for the eyes, others for the head; some for the teeth, others for the belly; and some for occult disorders. There were also physicians for female disorders. The sons followed the profession of their fathers, so that their number must necessarily have been very great. Herodotus says, παντα δι ιητρων ιατι πλια.* This arrangement and classification, however, could scarcely have taken place until the practice of

---

* ["Of physicians there are numbers."]

medicine had ceased with the priesthood. Such a distribution of practice might in cases where manual operation alone was required be attended with benefit; but with regard to cases in general, it would only serve to limit knowledge and confirm prejudice. The errors of the father would be transmitted to the son, and by him handed down to posterity. Confinement to one view and to one subject, of necessity incites quackery. Wherein consists the superiority of the regular practitioner over the empiric, but in the resources which his extended knowledge of the human frame and its function, enable him to apply? Every individual part is essentially connected with the whole — governed by the same laws, operated upon by the same influences and circumstances; nothing in the human body — either in health or disease — can, strictly speaking, be called local.

As the possession of medical knowledge was considered to be received through the direct agency of heaven, it is natural to conceive the exercise of it to have originated with the priests. In early and superstitious ages, as already shown, diseases were regarded as inflictions of the divine vengeance; and means were therefore sought to appease the anger of the gods, and mitigate the celestial wrath. Appeals to the oracles, divination, and magic, henceforth became connected with medicine. Hippocrates was the first physician to relieve medicine from the trammels of superstition and the delusions of philosophy.

Nothing could tend more to retard the progress of medicine, and paralyse all efforts for its improvement, than the opinion, once so generally entertained, of the celestial origin of disease, which, if admitted, appears necessarily to demand divine interposition for its relief. Religion and medicine were both brought into contempt by the adoption of sacrifices and incantations, and the mercenary practices of the priests to insure intercession with the gods. Hippocrates resisted this folly and wickedness, and boldly declared that no disease whatever came from the gods, but owed its origin to its own natural and manifest cause. Even the learned Celsus, whose works are universally read and admired at the present day, whose writings are considered as forming a conspicuous portion of our standard medical literature, was not free of the prejudices of his time, with regard to the origin of disease. In the preface to his work, 'De Re Medica,' he expressly says, "Morbos ad iram deorum immortalium relatos esse, et ab iisdem opem posci solitam."* He, however, had too much good sense not to rely upon remedies as his curative agents, and therefore, writes " Morbi, non eloquentia sed remediis curantur."

The religion of the ancient Egyptians was a kind of pantheism; they believed that the Divine Spirit was the soul of the world; yet some of their deities appear to have been worshipped by them and adored as supreme intelligences, whose notions were incomprehensible, but whose works were visible in the creation. The symbols by

---

* [Diseases are to be attributed to the anger of the immortal gods, and from them relief used to be sought.]

which their worship of the Deity in his works were at first acknowledged and reverenced, ceased in the course of time, under the general ignorance of the people, to be the types, and became the deities themselves.* The Egyptians divided the human body into thirty-six parts, each of which they believed to be under the particular government of one of the decans or aerial demons, who presided over the triple divisions of the twelve signs;† and we have the authority of Origen for saying, that when any part of the body was diseased, a cure was effected by invoking the demon to whose province it belonged. The late M. Champollion, whose services in the illustration of Egyptian antiquities and literature have been so distinguished, constructed a kind of theological anatomy out of the 'Great Funereal Ritual or Book of Manifestations.' This is frequently represented upon the mummy cases, but more particularly, either in

---

* See my Preliminary Essay to an intended Encyclopædia Ægyptiaca, London, 1842, 8vo., pp. 20, *et seq.*

† Concerning the decans, see Scaliger ad Manilium, Kircher II., parte Oedipi, Salmasius de Annis Climactericis, and Taylor's Notes on Jamblichus. Gale has also given a curious extract from Hermes relative to the same subject, which he derived from a MS. copy of Stobæus, which belonged to Vossius. Taylor has thus translated it: " We say, O son, that the body (of the universe) is comprehensive of all things. Conceive, therefore, this to be as it were of a circular form. But under the circle of this body the thirty-six decans are arranged, as the media of the whole circle of the zodiac. These likewise must be understood to preside as guardians over everything in the world, connecting and containing all things, and preserving the established order of all things, &c. They also possess, with respect to us, the greatest power."

whole or in part, in the papyri MSS.* Here, then, we see the first known attempt to assign the different parts of the body to the subjection of the different planets, which has been continued and handed down to us of the present day in the almanacs of the renowned astrologer and physician, Francis Moore.

How admirably and how humorously does Southey† describe the anatomy of man's body, as governed by zodiacal signs, and exhibited in that amusing work of the sixteenth century, the 'Margarita Philosophica'!

"There Homo stands, naked but not ashamed, upon the two Pisces, one foot upon each; the fish being neither in air, nor water, nor upon earth, but self-suspended as it appears in the void. Aries has alighted with two feet on Homo's head, and has sent a shaft through the forehead into his brain. Taurus has quietly seated himself across his neck. The Gemini are riding astride a little below his right shoulder. The whole trunk is laid open, as if part of the old accursed punishment for high treason had been performed upon him. The Lion occupies the thorax as his proper domain, and the Crab is in possession of the abdomen. Sagittarius, volant in the void, has just let fly an arrow, which is on the way to his right arm. Capricornus breathes out a visible influence that penetrates both knees; Aquarius inflicts

---

* For further information on this subject, see my History of Egyptian mummies. Lond. 1834, 4to., p. 148.

† Doctor, vol. iii., p. 112.

similar punctures upon both legs. Virgo fishes as it were at his intestines; Libra at the part affected by schoolmasters in their anger; and Scorpio takes the wickedest aim of all."

Manilius thus describes the appropriation of the zodiacal constellations to the various parts of man:

" Namque Aries capiti, Taurus cervicibus hæret;
Brachia sub Geminis consentur, pectora Cancro;
Te, scapulæ, Nemææ, vocant, teque ilia, Virgo;
Libra colit clunes, et Scorpius inguine regnat;
Et femur Arcitenens, genura et Capricornus amavit;
Cruraque defendit Juvenis, vestigia, Pisces."* †

The Egyptian Æsculapius must not be confounded with that of the Greeks. The mythological veil under which all traces of the history of the Egyptian medicine are to be found, serves only to demonstrate that the whole is to be looked upon as allegorical, as far as relates to the personages mentioned. The whole matter, as I have elsewhere shown,‡ reduces itself to fabulous history. Medicine, however, took its rise in the East, passed into Egypt, thence into Greece, and so was disseminated throughout the civilized world. All knowledge being in

* [The *Ram* claims the head; the *Bull* the neck; the twins the arms; the *Crab* the breast; the *Lion* the thorax; the *Virgin* the bowels; the *Scales* the reins; the *Scorpion* the secrets; the *Archer* the thighs; the *Goat* the knees; the *Water-carrier* the legs; and the *Fishes* the feet.]

† Astronomicon, lib. i.

‡ Memoir of Æsculapius in Medical Portrait Gallery, vol. i., p. 5.

the earliest times confined to the priests, and the art of healing being traced to a celestial origin, it is easy to comprehend its connexion with the ceremonials of religion, and in what manner, therefore, the superstitions, in relation to it, were cherished and monopolized by the priesthood. To their class application was of course made to invoke celestial aid, to appease the offended divinities, and to insure the restoration of health. Magic and divination were indeed looked upon as belonging to their sacred function, and regarded as the highest branches of the medical profession. " Magic, according to the Greeks," says Psellus,* "is a thing of a very powerful nature. They say that this forms the last part of the sacerdotal science. Magic, indeed investigates the nature, power, and quality of everything sublunary; viz., of the elements and their parts, of animals, all various plants and their fruits, of stones, and herbs; and, in short, it explores the essence and power of everything. From hence, therefore, it produces its effects. And it forms statues which procure health, makes all various figures, and things which become the instruments of disease. It asserts, too, that eagles and dragons contribute to health; but that cats, dogs, and crows, are symbols of vigilance, to which, therefore, they contribute. But for the fashioning of certain parts, wax and clay are used. Often, too, celestial fire is made

---

* In a rare Greek MS., on Dæmons according to the Dogmas of the Greeks; translated by T. Taylor. See his Jamblichus, p. 221, note.

to appear through magic; and these statues laugh, and lamps are spontaneously enkindled." The Council of Laodicea, A.D. 366, wisely forbade the priesthood the study and practice of enchantment, mathematics, astrology, and the binding of the soul by amulets.

There is reason to fear that the purposes of medicine were converted by the monks to the basest uses, and that the authority of the physician superadded to the terrors of the church, exercised over those in whom the mind was enfeebled by disease and incapable of exerting its power, were employed in the extortion of money and the indulgence of rapacity. Want of knowledge was supplied by mystery, and faith usurped the place of effectual proscription. Hence arose the employment of charms, amulets, relics, &c. The ignorance and the cupidity of the monks caused the Lateran Council, under the pontificate of Calistus II, A.D. 1123, to forbid the attendance of the priests and monks at the bedside of the sick, otherwise than as ministers of religion. Still, however, it was secretly followed, and Pope Innocent II, in a council at Rheims, A.D. 1131, enforced the decree prohibiting the monks frequenting schools of medicine, and directed them to confine their practice to the limits of their own monastery. Some, however, continued to pursue it, and some of the secular clergy practised it as generally as before, so that the decrees were found inefficient in the accomplishment of their object; and a Lateran Council, in A.D. 1139, threatened all who neglected its orders with the severest penalties and suspension from the exercise of all ecclesiasiltca functions; denouncing such practices as a neglect of the sacred objects of their profession in exchange for ungodly lucre. "Ordinis sui propositum nullatenus attendentes, pro *detestanda pecunia sanitatem pollicentes.*"*

When the priests ascer ained that they could no longer confine the practice of medicine to themselves it was stigmatized and denounced. At the Council of Tours, held in 1163 by Pope Alexander III., it was maintained that the devil, to seduce the priesthood from the duties of the altar, involved them in mundane occupations, which, under the plea of humanity, exposed them to constant and perilous temptations. They were accordingly prohibited the study of medicine, and that of the law, and every ecclesiastic who should infringe the decree was threatened with excommunication. In 1215 Pope Innocent III fulminated an anathema specially directed against surgery, by ordaining, that as the church abhorred all cruel or sanguinary practices, no priest should be permitted to follow surgery, or to perform any operations in which either instruments of steel or fire were employed; and that they should refuse their benediction to all those who professed and pursued it.

Stringent as these measures were, they were found inadequate to effect the purpose intended, and it was only at length accomplished by a special bull procured from the Pope, which, by

---

* [Not attending to the object of their order, promising health for filthy lucre.]

permitting physicians to marry, effectually divorced medicine from theology.

In many catholic countries, however, the saints have proved sad enemies to the doctors.* Miraculous cures are attested by monks, abbots,

* The priests, in some parts of Italy, still hold their medical influence. An ingenious young physician, travelling in that country in 1838, met with several instances during his stay in Naples. In one case he was asked by the parents of a poor girl to visit their child who was ill of a fever. He accompanied them to their miserable cabin, and found her in an advanced stage of typhus, yet not, he thought, hopelessly beyond the reach of art. He prescribed for her, and laid down strict injunctions to be followed during his absence. Upon visiting her again, he was surprised to find that his directions had not been followed, nor the treatment he directed pursued. She was now *in articulo mortis*. As he had not intruded his advice, this conduct on the part of the parents at first seemed inexplicable; but he soon found an explanation in the appearance of a priest, who, regardless of his presence, advanced to the bedside, and, inquiring whether his medicine had been administered, unfolded a paper containing a black salve, a minute portion of which he placed upon her tongue, and then harangued in a most intemperate manner upon the abomination the parents had been guilty of in seeking assistance from a heretic, who, he said, would be sure to administer poison in place of balm to their ills. In other cases the physician met with similar conduct.

At the time of the prevalence of the cholera in Canada, a man named Ayres, who came out of the States, and was said to be a graduate of the University of New Jersey, was given out to be St. Roche, the principal patron saint of the Canadians, and renowned for his power in averting pestilential diseases. He was reported to have descended from heaven to cure his suffering people of the cholera, and many were the cases in which he appeared to afford relief. Many were thus dispossessed of their fright in anticipation of the disease, who might, probably, but for his inspiriting influence, have fallen victims to their apprehensions. The remedy he employed was an admixture of maple sugar, charcoal, and lard.

bishops, popes, and consecrated saints. St. Martin's shrine alone is said to have restored fifty blind people to the blessing of sight; stories related no less at variance with the sentiments and characters of the men than contradicted by the laws of nature. Pilgrimages and visits to holy shrines have usurped the place of medicine, and, as in many cases at our own watering places, by air and exercise, have unquestionably effected what the employment of regular professional aid had been unable to accomplish. St. Dominic, St. Bellinus, and St. Vitus have been greatly renowned in the cure of diseases in general; the latter particularly, who takes both poisons and madness of all kinds under his special protection.

Melton* says " the saints of the Romanists have usurped the place of the zodiacal constellations in their governance of the parts of man's body, and that 'for every limbe they have a saint.' Thus St. Otilia keepes the head instead of Aries; St. Blasius is appointed to governe the necke instead of Taurus; St. Lawrence keepes the backe and shoulders instead of Gemini, Cancer, and Leo; St. Erasmus rules the belly with the entrayles, in the place of Libra and Scorpius; in the stead of Sagittarius, Capricornus, Aquarius, and Pisces, the holy church of Rome hath elected St. Burgarde, St. Rochus, St. Quirinus, St. John, and many others, which governe the thighs, feet, shinnes, and knees."

This supposed influence of the Romish saints

---

* Astrologaster, p. 20.

is more minutely exhibited, according to Hone, in two very old prints, from engravings on wood, in the collection of the British Museum. *Right hand:* the top joint of the thumb is dedicated to God, the second joint to the Virgin; the top joint of the fore-finger to St. Barnabas, the second joint to St. John, the third to St. Paul; the top joint of the second finger to Simon Cleophas, the second joint to Tathideo, the third to Joseph; the top joint of the third finger to Zaccheus, the second to Stephen, the third to the evangelist Luke; the top-joint of the little finger to Leatus, the second to Mark, the third to Nicodemus. *Left hand:* the top joint of the thumb is dedicated to Christ, the second joint to the Virgin; the top joint of the fore-finger to St. James, the second to St. John the Evangelist, the third to St. Peter: the first joint of the second finger to St. Simon, the second joint to St. Matthew, the third to St. James the Great; the top joint of the third finger to St. Jude, the second joint to St. Bartholomew, the third to St. Andrew; the top joint of the little finger to St. Matthias, the second joint to St. Thomas, the third joint to St. Philip.

The following list, though doubtless very imperfect, will yet serve to show how general was the appropriation of particular diseases to the Roman Catholic saints:

St. Agatha, against sore breasts.
St. Agnan and St. Tignan, against scald head.
St. Anthony, against inflammations.

St. Apollonia, against toothache.
St. Avertin, against lunacy.
St. Benedict, against the stone, and also for poisons.
St. Blaise, against the quinsey, bones sticking in the throat, &c.
St. Christopher and St. Mark, against sudden death.
St. Clara against sore eyes.
St. Erasmus against the colic.
St. Eutrope, against dropsy.
St. Genow and St. Maur, against the gout.
St. Germanus, against the diseases of children.
St. Giles and St. Hyacinth, against sterility.
St. Herbert, against hydrophobia.
St. Job and St. Fiage, against syphilis.
St. John, against epilepsy and poison.
St. Lawrence, against diseases of the back and shoulders.
St. Liberius, against the stone and fistula.
St. Maine, against the scab.
St. Margaret and St. Edine, against danger in parturition.
St. Martin, against the itch.
St. Marus, against palsy and convulsions.
St. Otilia and St. Juliana, against sore eyes and the headache.
St. Pernel, against the ague.
St. Petronilla, St. Apollonia, and St. Lucy, against the toothache.
——————, and St. Genevieve, against fevers.
St. Phaire, against hemorrhoids.
St. Quintan, against coughs.

St. Rochus, and St. Sebastian, against the plague.
St. Romanus, against demoniacal possession.
St. Ruffin, against madness.
St. Sigismund, against fevers and agues.
St. Valentin, against epilepsy.
St. Venise, against chlorosis.
St. Vitus, against madness and poisons.
St. Wallia and St. Wallery, against the stone.
St. Wolfgang, against lameness.

Many wells and fountains have various virtues and superstitions attached to them. Those which are medicinal are generally named after some patron saint. To these pilgrims resorted, and also the sick, for relief from their diseases. They were called holy wells, or holy springs, wishing wells, &c., and various rites were performed at them at Easter, upon holy Thursday, and other particular days. Offerings were made to propitiate, or to obtain the favour of the patron saint, and among the rest a custom was very prevalent to deposit rags. Grose, from a MS. in the Cotton Library, (Julius F. 6,) tells us that "between the towns of Alton and Newton, near the foot of Rosberrye Toppinge, there is a well dedicated to St. Oswald. The neighbours have an opinion that a shirt taken off a sick person and thrown into that well will show whether the person will recover or die: for, if it floated, it denoted the recovery of the party; if it sunk, there remained no hope of their life: and to reward the saint for his intelligence, they *tear off a rag of the shirt, and leave it hanging on the briars thereabouts:* "where," says the writer, "I have seen such numbers as might have made a fayre rheme in a paper-myll." Pennant, Heron (Pinkerton), Sinclair, Macaulay, Brand, and many other authors relate similar practices in different parts of the world. The kingdom of Ireland affords numerous examples of the superstitions entertained with regard to the miraculous power of certain fountains, holy wells, &c. Many a tedious and wearisome journey has been made to some specified place for the obtaining of health, as well as a penance for sins. Mr. and Mrs. Hall, in their very interesting and faithful work on Ireland,* tells us that sanctified wells are to be found in nearly all the parishes of the kingdom. They are generally betokened by the erection of rude crosses immediately above them, by fragments of cloth, and bits of rags of all colours, hung upon the neighbouring bushes and left as memorials; sometimes the crutches of convalescent visitors are bequeathed as offerings, and not unfrequently small buildings, for prayer and shelter, have been raised above and around them. Each holy well has its stated day, when a pilgrimage is supposed to be peculiarly fortunate; the patron day, *i. e.*, the day of its patron saint, attracts crowds of visitors, some with the hope of receiving health from its waters, others as a place of meeting with distant friends; but the great majority of them are lured into the neighbourhood by a love of idleness and dissipation. The scene therefore is, or rather was, disgusting to

* Vol. i., p. 280.

a degree; but the evil has of late greatly diminished; and, since the spread of temperance, there being neither drinking nor fighting in the vicinity, the attendants are almost entirely limited to the holiday-keepers and the credulous.

At St. Ronague's well, a few miles distant from Cork, where numbers had assembled to receive the benefits of the water, the authorities I have just referred to say, "two old women were dipping up the water in tin cans, and exchanging supplies for small coins from the applicants; and when they had filled their bottles (brought for the purpose), and knelt at the rude cross, and repeated a few 'paters' and 'aves' before it, they departed to their homes in peace and quietness; the only objects worthy of remark connected with the ceremony being two or three blind pilgrims, who stood by the sides of the well and handed to each comer a thin pebble, with which he signed the mark of the cross upon a large stone at the well head, and which frequent rubbing had deeply indented."

The holy well, Tubber Quan, near Carrick-on-Suir, is in great repute for the many miraculous cures effected by its waters. The well, we learn,* is dedicated to two patron saints, St. Quan, after whom it takes its name, and St. Brogawn. The times for visiting it are the last three Sundays in June, when the people imagine the saints exert their sacred influence more particularly for the benefit of those who apply for their assistance. It is confidently said, and

---

* Ibid., p. 281.

firmly believed, that at this period the two saints appear in the well in the shape of two small fishes, of the trout kind; and if they do not so appear, that no cures will take place. The penitents attending on these occasions ascend the hill barefoot, kneel by the stream and repeat a number of paters and aves, then enter it, go through the stream three times, at a slow pace, reciting their prayers. They then go on the gravel-walk, and traverse it round three times on their bare knees, often till the blood starts in the operation, repeat their prayers, then traverse three times round a tree on their bare knees, but upon the grass. Having performed these exercises they cut off locks of their hair and tie them on the branches of the tree as specifics against headache. The tree is a great object of veneration, and presents a curious spectacle, being covered all over with human hair.

Bishop Hall records a miraculous cure effected on a man by washing in St. Madern's Well in Cornwall, to which he was three times admonished in a dream. Father Francis gives a particular account of the same case. The holy well at Basingwerk, celebrated by Ranulf Higden in his Polychronicon, was a spring of great celebrity for its wonderful cures. Pilgrims resorted to it to pay their devotions. The stones about it were marked with red streaks, being symbols of the blood of St. Wenefride martyred by Caradoc.

Mr. Robert Kier, of Falkirk, a correspondent of the editor of the 'Every Day Book,' mentions the visiting of certain wells supposed to have healing properties in the month of May, as among the superstitions of the Scotch; and in the Sessions Records, (June 12, 1628,) it is reported that a number of persons were brought before the Kirk Session of Falkirk, accused of going to Christ's Well on the Sundays of May to seek their health, and the whole being found guilty were sentenced to repent "in linens" three several sabbaths. In 1657 a number of persons were publicly rebuked for visiting the well of Airth. The custom was to leave a piece of money and a napkin at the well, from which they took a can of the water, and were not to speak a word either in going or returning, nor on any account to spill a drop of the water. Notwithstanding these proceedings, many are known to have lately travelled several miles into the Highlands, there to obtain water for the cure of their sick cattle.

The relics belonging to saints have been esteemed of equal efficiency in removing diseases: the belt of St. Guthlac, and the felt of St. Thomas of Lancaster, were sovereign remedies for the headache, whilst the penknife and boots of Archbishop Becket, and a piece of his shirt, were found most admirably to aid parturition.

TALISMANS.

"Old wives and starres are his counsellers: his night-spell is his guard, and charms his physicians. He wears Paracelsian characters for the toothache; and a little hallowed wax is his antidote for all evils."

Bishop Hall.

I HAVE already alluded to the probable origin of Talismans from the belief that certain substances are externally impressed with the characters of their properties and virtues by the influence of the planetary bodies. A talisman may, in general terms, be defined to be a substance composed of certain cabalistical characters engraved on stone, metal, or other material, or else written on slips of paper. It differs from an amulet in this respect, that it may be deposited in any place, or carried about the person without losing its efficacy, whilst the latter requires to be constantly worn about the individual. Dr. Hyde[*] quotes a Persian writer, who defines the Telesm or Talisman to be "a piece of art compounded of the celestial powers and elementary bodies, appropriated to certain figures and positions, and purposes, and times, contrary to the usual manner;" and Maimonides[†] remarks that

---

[*] Syntagma, a Greg. Sharpe, vol. i., p. 500.
[†] More Nevochim, part i., cap. l., p. 2.

images or idols were called *Tzelamim,* not from their figure or form, but from the power or influence which was supposed to reside in them. The Rev. Mr. Townley* has suggested that the first construction of astrological or talismanic images probably arose from the desire of idolaters to represent the planets during their absence from the horizon, so that they might at all times be able to worship either the planetary body itself, or its representative. The astrologers, therefore, appropriated particular colours, metals, stones, trees, &c., to the respective planets they designed to represent, and constructed them when the planets were in their exaltation, and in a happy conjunction with other heavenly bodies; after which they attempted by incantatory rites, to inspire the fabricated symbols with the power and influence of the planets themselves.†

The Hebrew word for talisman (magan) signifies a paper or other material, drawn or engraved with the letters composing the sacred name JEHOVAH, or with other characters, and improperly applied to astrological representations, because, like the letters composing " The Incommunicable Name," they were supposed to serve as a defence against sickness, lightning, and tempest.‡ It was a common practice with magicians, whenever a plague or other great calamity infested a country, to make a supposed

* The Reasons of the Laws of Moses, p. 113.

† See Pocockii Spec. Hist. Arab., p. 140. Hyde de Vet. Pers. Relig., cap. v., p. 126. Young on Idolatrous Corruptions, vol. i., p. 113.

‡ Gaffarel, Curiositez Inouyes, cap. vi., p. 106.

image of the destroyer, either in gold, silver, clay, wax, &c., under a certain configuration of the heavens, and to set it up in some particular place that the evil might be stayed.

Talisman are of various kinds. Fosbrooke* has arranged them into five divisions:—1. The *Astronomical*, with celestial signs and intelligible characters. 2. The *Magical*, with extraordinary figures, superstitious words, and names of unknown angels. 3. The *Mixed*, of celestial signs and barbarous words, but not superstitious, or with names of angels. 4. The *Sigilla Planetarum*, composed of Hebrew numeral letters, used by astrologers and fortune-tellers. 5. *Hebrew Names and Characters*. These were formed according to the cabalistic art.

A Hebrew talisman is given in the 'Gentleman's Magazine,'† which reads: " It overflowed — he did cast darts — Shadai is all sufficient — his hand is strong, and is the preserver of my life in all its variations."

The Phylacteries (of which I have elsewhere given a particular account)‡ ought properly to be regarded as talismans, rather than amulets. They are of three kinds, and used for the head, the arm, and also attached to the door-posts. Upon these, various portions of Holy Writ are inscribed, and they are directed to be prepared in a peculiar manner.

Amulets in the form of inscriptions are called

---

* Encyclopædia of Antiquities, vol. i., p. 336.
† Vol. lviii., pp. 586, 695.
‡ Bibliotheca Sussexiana, vol. i., part i., pp. xxxvi-viii.

Characts. From Arnot's 'History of Edinburgh,' we learn that "on all the old houses still existing in Edinburgh, there are remains of talismanic or cabalistical characters, which the superstition of earlier ages had caused to be engraved on their fronts. These were generally composed of some text of Scripture of the name of God, or, perhaps, of an emblematic representation of the resurrection."

AMULETS.

"When time shall once have laid his lenient hand on the passions and pursuits of the present moment, they too shall lose that imaginary value which heated fancy now bestows upon them." BLAIR.

In Arabic the word Amulet means "that which is suspended." It has been said to be derived from the barbarous Latin word amuletum, from amolior, to remove, (*a* and *moles*, a heap or mass, to heave away, to drive away, to repel,) also from amula, a small vessel with lustral water in it, which the Romans frequently carried in their pockets for purification and expiation; and according to Pliny, many were made in the shape of little vessels, carved out of a piece of amber, and hung about the children's necks. But there is little doubt of its eastern origin.

A belief in the efficacy of an amulet or charm to ward off diseases, to avert contagion, and infection from diseases whose origin is most obscure and whose extent is most indefinite, to cure diseases when imbibed or existing, to protect against supernatural agency, the evil eye, magical arts, divination, sorcery, &c., has prevailed from a very early time. The use of amulets was common among the Greeks and the Romans, whose amulets were principally formed of gems, crowns of pearls, necklaces of coral, shells, &c. The Athletæ wore amulets to ensure to themselves victory: they were suspended from the neck. The power of amulets was in former times considered so effectual that Grose tells us an oath was administered to persons going to fight a legal duel "that they had ne charme ne herb of virtue." St. Chrysostom and other of the fathers are loud in their condemnation of the practice.

In its composition the amulet is of the most varied kinds; objects selected either from the animal, the vegetable, or the mineral kingdoms; pieces of old rags or garments, scraps of writing in legible or illegible characters, in fact, of anything to which any superstitious property has been considered to belong. Sir Walter Scott had in his possession one of these pretended charms taken from an old woman who was said to charm and injure her neighbours' cattle. It consisted of feathers, parings of nails, hair, and such like trash, wrapped in a lump of clay. The amulets of the Chaldeans and Persians were generally made in a cylindrical form, and had by their figures and characters an astrological import, and it is not improbable but that they consisted of the horoscope of the possessor.

> "Of talismans and sigils knew the power,
> And carefully watch'd the planetary hour."
> Pope.

Count Caylus, D'Olivier, Millin, and other

ingenious antiquaries have looked upon the ancient Babylonian cylinders as amulets; but Landseer* has shown that, according to the manner in which they are engraved, being in intaglio, they were well fitted to be used as seals. In the East, generally, the amulet consists of certain names of the Deity, verses of the Koran, or particular passages compressed into a very small space, rolled up, and are to be found concealed in the shash of the turban. The Christians wore amulets with verses selected from the Old or New Testament, and particularly from the Gospel of St. John. The amulets or charms called *grigris* by the African priests are of a similar description. A considerable traffic was carried on, according to Barbot and other travellers,† in vending these pretended preservatives against thunderbolts and diseases, to procure many wives and to give to them easy deliveries, to avert shipwreck or slavery, and to secure victory in battle. One, destined to the latter purpose, was in the museum of Sir Ashton Lever, which had belonged to a king of Brak, in Senegal, who, however, had the misfortune to be killed in battle with the charm upon him. It formed a fine chaplet for the head, to which it was attached with many-coloured bands. The rolled paper contained within it had the following sentences from the Koran:

"In the name of the merciful God! Pray to God through our Lord Mohammed.

---

* Sabæan Researches, p. 58.
† In Churchill's Collection of Voyages, vol. v., pp. 60 and 104.

"All that exists is so only by his command. He gives life, and also calls sinners to an account. He deprives us of life by the sole power of his name: these are undeniable truths. He that lives owes his life to the peculiar clemency of his Lord, who by his providence takes care of his subsistence. He is a wise prince or governor."

Other grigris have been found to contain other parts of the Koran.

From mere sentences or arrangement of words peculiar substances came to be employed, and are employed even to this day; in this country sometimes under a presumed efficacy or virtue in the substance itself, free of any superstitious spell as to the mode of its application, as in the use of camphor worn about the person to avert febrile contagion, anodyne necklaces to assist in dentition, &c.

Amulets are frequently met with composed of various stones carved or fashioned into a particular shape, representing an animal or other object. These, singly or associated together, are strung into necklaces and worn round the neck, wrist, or other part of the body. The necklaces so commonly found on the Egyptian mummies are usually composed of objects having a funereal or mythological character or import, and were doubtless used as amulets to preserve the integrity of the body — a circumstance peculiarly essential with the Egyptians, being in accordance with their system of theology.

Precious stones were often employed as amulets; and some, not content to wear them externally, adopted the means of reducing them to powder, and taking them as internal remedies. Lapis Armenus, an ochre of copper, of a dark blue colour, and Lapis lazuli (azure stone), are extolled by Alexander, Ætius, Avicenna, and Actuarius as sovereign remedies for melancholy when taken internally. Butler quotes from Encelius, who says that the garnet, if hung about the neck or taken in drink, much assisteth sorrow and recreates the heart; and the chrysolite is described as the friend of wisdom and the enemy to folly. *Inducit sapientiam fugat stultitiam.** Renodeus admires precious stones because they adorn king's crowns, grace the fingers, enrich our household stuff, defend us from enchantments, preserve health, cure diseases, drive away grief, cares, and exhilarate the mind. "Regum coronas ornant, digitos illustrant, supellectilem ditant, è fascino, tuentur, morbis medentur, sanitatem conservant, mortem exhilarant, tristitiam pellunt."†

"Heliotropius stauncheth blood, driveth away poisons, preserveth health; yea, and some write that it provoketh raine, and darkeneth the sunne, suffering not him that beareth it to be abused."‡

"A topaze healeth the lunaticke person of his passion of lunacie."§

"Corneolus (cornelian) mitigateth the heate of the minde and qualifieth malice, it stancheth bloodie fluxes."‖

---

* [It brings wisdom and expels folly.]
† Præfat. ad Lap. Prec., lib. ii., sect. 2, de Mat. Med.
‡ Reg. Scot.   § Ibid.   ‖ Ibid.

AMULETS.

"A sapphire preserveth the members and maketh them livelie, and helpeth agues and gowts, and suffereth not the bearer to be afraid; it hath virtue against venome, and staieth bleeding at the nose, being often put thereto."*

Precious metals as well as precious stones, administered internally, are of renowned efficacy. Chaucer says,

> "For gold in physick is a cordial,
> Therefore he loved gold in special."

The Mischna permits the Jews to wear amulets provided they have been found efficacious in at least three cases by an approved person.

Odd numbers† have always been regarded as of serious import. They often form charms and are applied to physic. Ravenscroft, in his comedy of 'Mammamouchi, or the Citizen turned Gentleman,' makes Trickmore as a physician to say, " Let the number of his bleedings and purgations be odd, *numero Deus impare gaudet.*"‡ Every one knows that the seventh son of a seventh son is an infallible doctor. "The

---

* Ibid.

† Among my extracts from ancient writers, I find the following, but do not recollect whence it was taken: "Some philosophers are of opinion that all things are composed of number, prefer the odd before the other, and attribute to it a great efficacy and perfection, especially in matters of physic: wherefore it is that many doctors prescribe always an odd pill, an odd draught, or drop to be taken by their patients. For the perfection thereof they allege these following numbers: as 7 Planets, 7 wonders of the World, 9 Muses, 3 Graces, God is 3 in 1, &c."

‡ [God delights in an odd number.]

seventh son of a seventh son is born a physician; having an intuitive knowledge of the art of curing all disorders, and sometimes the faculty of performing wonderful cures by touching only."* M. Thiers† reasons the point: "Plusieurs croyent qu'en France, les septièmes garçons, nez de legitimes mariages, sans que la suitte des sept ait, esté interrompue par la naissance d'aucune fille, peuvent aussi guerir des fièvres tierces, des fièvres quartes, et mesme des ecrouelles, après avoir jeûné trois ou neuf jours avant que de toucher les malades. Mais ils font trop de fond sur le nombre septenaire, en attribuant au septième garçon, preferablement à tous autres, une puissance qu'il y a autant de raison d'attribuer au sixième ou au huitième, sur le nombre de trois, et sur celuy de neuf, pour ne pas s'engager dans la superstition. Joint que de trois que je connois de ces septièmes garçons il y en a deux qui ne guerissent de rien, et que le troisième m'a avoué de bonne foy, qu'il avoit en autrefois la reputation de guerir de quantité des maux, quoique en effet il n'ait jamais guery d'aucun. C'est pourquoy Monsieur du Laurent a grande raison de rejetter ce pretendu pouvoir, et de la mettre au rang des fables, en ce qui concerne la guerison des ecrouelles."‡

* MS. Julius F. 6, Cotton Library.
† Traité des Superstitions, p. 436.
‡ [Many believe, in France, that the sevenths sons born in lawful marriage, if no girl comes between, can cure tertians, quartans, and even the King's evil, provided they fast three or nine days before touching those afflicted. But they reckon too much on the seventh number, when they attribute to the

ABRAXAS. The origin of this word is obscure. It denotes a power presiding over 365 others, and corresponds with the number of days in the year. It is of Egyptian origin, but it can be technically explained by certain Greek letters used as equivalents for numbers: thus, A 1, B 2, P 100, A 1, Ξ 60, Σ 200, which make 365. It is spelt in this way by all the Greek fathers. Beausobre derives the word from the two Greek words which signify "Magnificent Saviour," αβρος and Σαω. It formed a symbol employed by the heresiarch Basilides, who was accused by the fathers of magic, and who certainly promulgated many superstitions. His abraxas consisted of a small figure as a talisman, which he regarded as the representative of the Prince of the Eons, or the 365 heavens, or rather angels belonging to these heavens. By this figure, however, the Egyptians had previously professed to dispossess evil spirits and also to cure diseases. It is therefore borrowed by Basilides of these people. Chifflet, Montfaucon, and others have figured many of the abraxas. The engraved gems which have the word abraxas impressed upon them, and sometimes also a symbol, or the latter without the word, are called abraxas, and

seventh child, in preference to all the rest, a power which they might as well ascribe to the sixth or eighth. Of three of these seventh sons that I know, there are two who cure nobody, and the third has confessed to me that he once enjoyed the reputation of being able to cure numerous diseases, although he had never cured any. Consequently, M. du Laurent has good reason to reject this visionary power, and place this method of curing the King's evil in the rank of fables.]

used as amulets against diseases. The learned Lardner* treats extensively on this subject. He particularly notices the extraordinary collection given by Montfaucon; and he concludes that they are "too numerous, too costly, and too heathenish to be remains of any Christian sect." The materials are costly, and they have figures of the cock, dog, lion, ape, sphynx, Isis, Osiris, Serapis, Harpocrates, Canopus, the scarabæus, &c. St. Jerome makes abraxas to be the same as mythras, which is a Persian deity and known to be the sun. Abraxas may therefore be considered as presiding over the 365 heavens, as the sun is the ruler of the day, and the year consists of 365 days. Apollo and the sun in ancient mythology are the same, and Apollo was the god of physic or healing — the sense in which these abraxæi were employed.

Peculiar arrangements of words and letters, as well as numbers, also constituted amulets.

ABRACADABRA or ABRASADABRA. This magical word is recommended on the authority of Serenus Samonicus, a physician in the reign of Caracalla, as a charm or amulet to cure ague and other diseases:

"Mortiferum magis est, quod Græcis hemitritæum†
Vulgatur verbis, hoc nostra dicere lingua

---

* Works, vol. ix., pp. 290-364.

† [What the Greeks call hemitritæum (ague) is still more fatal. We have no word for it in our (the Latin) language. Write the word Abracatabra on a slip of paper, cutting off the first and last letters in every succeeding line till the word ends in a point. Remember to fasten it round your neck, &c.]

AMULETS.

Non potuere ulli, puto, nec voluere parentes.
Inscribis chartæ, quod dicitur Abracatabra,
Sæpius et subter repetis, sed detrahe summam,
Et magis atque magis desint elementa figuris
Singula, quæ semper rapies, et cætera figes,
Donec in angustum redigatur litera conum
His lino nexis collum redimire memento," &c.*

The letters comprising Abracadabra are to be so written, that reading from the apex on the right and up the left side, the same word will be given as at the top:

ABRACADABRA
BRACADABR
RACADAB
ACADA
CAD
A

or thus:

ABRACATABRA
ABRACATABR
ABRACATAB
ABRACATA
ABRACAT
ABRACA
ABRAC
ABRA
ABR
AB
A

Julius Africanus says, that pronouncing the

---

* Quint. Se. Samon. de Medic. Tiguri, 1540, cap. li., p. 224.

word in the same manner will be equally efficacious as writing it. Abracadabra was a god, and worshipped as such by the Tyrians. The Jews attributed an equal virtue to the word Aracalan employed in the same way.

CHARMS.

"Such medicines are to be exploded that consist of words, characters, spells, and charms, which can do no good at all, but out of a strong conceit, as Pomponatius proves; or the Devil's policy, who is the first founder and teacher of them."
BURTON.

CHARMS and Amulets have a similar signification and imply a similarity of power, the difference consisting rather in the manner in which they are severally used, than in any difference of their nature. Amulets were to be suspended when employed, charms are not necessarily subjected to such a method of application. The word charm is derived from the Latin word Carmen, signifying a verse in which the spells were very commonly but not uniformly written, and supposed to work their magical power. Some of these come properly under the head of exorcism or incantations, as that most ancient one handed down to us by Cato the Censor, who gives the following for the reduction of a dislocated limb:

"Luxum si quod est hac cantione sanum fiet, harundinem prende tibi viridem P. IIII. aut V longam. Mediam diffinde, et duo homines teneant ad coxendices. Incipe cantare IN ALIO S. F. MOTAS VAETA, DARIES DARDARIES ASTATARIES DISSUNAPITUR, usque dum coeant. Ferrum insuper jactato ubi coierint, et altera alteram tetigerit, id manu prende, et dextra sinistra præcide. Ad luxum, aut ad fracturam alliga, sanum fiet, et tamen quotidie cantato in alio S. F. vel luxato. Vel hoc modo, HUAT HANAT ISTA PISTA SISTA, DOMIABO DAMNAUSTRA, et luxato. Vel hoc modo, HUAT HAUT HAUT ISTA SIS TAR SIS ARDAUNABON DAMNAUSTRA."* †

There is scarcely a disease for which a charm has not been given, and I shall presently narrate some of the principal ones; and by classing them according to the disorders for which they have been recommended and employed, it will be seen that they apply principally to derangements of the nervous system, or to those diseases which are periodical in their character, and known by physicians to be especially subject to the influence of the passions and the emotions of the mind in general.

But it is not only to diseases of the body and mind to which they were directed to be applied; charms were also employed to avert evil, and counteract supposed malignant influences.

Thus among the natives of the Eastern Islands, an opinion long prevailed that by the use of amulets, the wearer would be rendered

---

* De Re Rustica, ed. Schneideri. Lips. 1794. CLX.-LXI.

† [A dislocation may be cured by this charm. Take a reed four or five feet long; cut it in the middle, and let two men hold the points towards each other for insertion. While this is doing, repeat these words: "IN ALIO S. F. MOTAS .... &c. Now jerk a piece of iron upon the reeds at their juncture, and cut right and left. Bind them to the dislocation or fracture, and it will effect a cure, &c.]

invulnerable. De Barros, the historian, says, that the Portuguese in vain attempted to destroy a Malay so long as he wore a bracelet containing a bone set in gold, which rendered him proof against their swords. This amulet was afterwards transmitted to the Viceroy Affonso d'Alboquerque, as a valuable present.

In the travels of Marco Polo, we read that in an attempt by Kublai Khan to make a conquest of the island of Zipangu, a jealousy arose between the two commanders of the exhibition, which led to an order for putting the whole of the inhabitants of the garrison to the sword; and that in obedience thereto, the heads of all were cut off, excepting of eight persons, who, by the efficacy of a diabolical charm, consisting of a jewel or amulet introduced into the right arm, between the skin and the flesh, were rendered secure from the effects of iron, either to kill or wound. Upon this discovery being made, they were beaten with a heavy wooden club, and presently died.*

The practice of physic among the Sumatrans is carried on by old men and women, and they generally procure a small sum in advance from their patients, under the pretext of purchasing charms. These are hung about the necks of children, and also worn by persons who are exposed to risk. They consist of long narrow scrolls of paper filled with incoherent scraps of verse, which are separated from each other by fanciful

* Travels of Marco Polo, translated by W. Marsden. Lond. 1818, 4to., p. 570.

drawings. Mr. Marsden accidentally met with one given for the ague. It was as follows: "(Sign of the cross.) When Christ saw the cross he trembled and shaked: and they said unto him, hast thou the ague? and he said unto them, I have neither ague nor fever; and whosoever bears these words, either in writing or in mind, shall never be troubled with ague or fever. So help thy servants, O Lord, who put their trust in thee!"*

In the account of Sungei-tenang country, Mr. Marsden relates that the people commonly carry charms about their persons to preserve them from accidents; one of which, printed at Batavia or Samarang in Java in Dutch, Portuguese, and French, was shown to him. It purported that the writer was acquainted with the occult sciences, and that whoever possessed one of the papers impressed with his mark (which was the figure of a hand with the thumb and fingers extended) was invulnerable and free from all kinds of harm.†

William Jackson, a Roman Catholic and a proscribed smuggler, was tried for and convicted of murder at Chichester, in January 1748–9, and sentence of death was passed upon him, and he was directed to be hung in chains. He however died in gaol a few hours after the sentence had been delivered. Upon being measured for his chains, in a linen purse upon his person was found the following charm:

---

* Hist. of Sumatra, p. 189.
† Ibid., p. 323.

CHARMS.

"Sancti tres Reges
Gaspar, Melchior, Balthasar,
Orate pro nobis nunc et in hora
Mortis nostræ."*

"Ces billets ont touche aux trois testes de S. S. Roys à Cologne. Ils sont pour les voyagers, contre les malheurs de chemins, maux de teste, mal-caduque, fièvres, sorcellerie, toute sorte de malefice, mort subite."† ‡

The Orientals generally have a belief in the influence of what is called "The Evil Eye," to the operation of which children are supposed to be the most susceptible: to avert the consequences, they are furnished with charms of various kinds. As an amulet against Fascination in general, but more particularly against the Evil Eye, Mr. Douce tells us§ that certain figures in bronze, coral, ivory, &c., representing a closed hand with the thumb thrust out between the first and second fingers called the *fig*, were common. In Henry IV., Part ii., Pistol says:

"When Pistol lies, do this; and fig me, like
The bragging Spaniard."

---

* "Ye three sacred kings
Gaspar, Melchior, Balthusar,
Pray for us now, and in the hour
Of our death.

† Gents. Mag., vol. xix., p. 88.

‡ [These papers are impressed three times with the mark of S. S. Royas of Cologne. They are intended for travellers, against the dangers of travelling, epilepsy, fevers, witchcraft, all kinds of spells, and sudden death.]

§ Illustrations of Shakspeare, vol. i., p. 493.

Coral is a substance which was generally considered to possess the power of keeping off evil spirits and averting the baneful consequences of the Evil Eye. Paracelsus recommends it to be worn round the necks of children as a remedy against fits, sorcery, charms, and poisons. Levinus Lemnius says, "Corall bound to the neck takes off turbulent dreams and allays the nightly fears of children. It preserveth such as bear it from fascination or bewitching, and in this respect is hanged about children's necks." The bells affixed to the coral toy with which children used formerly to be generally arrayed, have been conjectured to have been attached for the same purpose, as the ringing or rattling of them have been esteemed inimical to witches, sorcerers, &c.

Charms and incantations were common among the Druids for the cure of disease. According to Lord Northampton* the charm used by Mother Joane of Stowe to cure beastes, or men and women from diseases, was as follows:

> " Our Lord was the fyrst Man,
> That ever thorne prick't upon:
> It never blysted nor it never belted,
> And I pray God, nor this not may."

Rags, old clothes, pins and needles are frequent objects employed as charms. They are prevalent in the east as well as in Europe and England. In Persia they are common, and there exists a general superstition that to relieve disease or accident, the patient has only to de-

---

* Defensative against the Poyson of supposed Prophecies. Lond. 1583, 4to.

posit a rag on certain bushes, and from the same spot to take another which has been previously left from the same motive by a former sufferer.* The bushes in the neighbourhood of the Holy Wells attest the same practice. In Grand Cairo, pieces of garments that have touched the pilgrim camel, which carries the Grand Seignior's annual present, are preserved with great veneration, and when any of their families lie dangerously ill, they lay these things upon their bodies as infallible remedies.†

Having thus far treated of Talismans, Amulets, and Charms in general, and their employment in the cure of diseases and the averting of danger, I shall now proceed to specify some of the particular disorders to which they have been generally considered as most applicable.

Epilepsy, Convulsions, and Fits. The Elder Tree, to the history of which many superstitions belong, forms a charm for a variety of diseases, but has been especially employed in epilepsy. In Blochwick's 'Anatomie of the Elder,' translated and published, Lond. 1655, p. 52, we read of an amulet made of the elder growing on a Sallow: "If in the month of October, a little before the full moon, you pluck a twig of the elder, and cut the cane that is betwixt two of its knees, or knots, in nine pieces, and these pieces being bound in a piece of linen, be in a thread, so hung about the neck, that they touch the spoon of the heart, or the sword-formed carti-

---

* Morier's Journey to Persia, p. 230.
† Haynes's Letters, No. 7, p. 90.

lage; and that they may stay more firmly in that place, they are to be bound thereon with a linen or silken roller wrapt about the body, till the thread break of itself. The thread being broken and the roller removed, the amulet is not at all to be touched with bare hands, but it ought to be taken hold on by some instrument and buried in a place that nobody may touch it."

Some hang a cross made of the elder and the sallow, mutually inwrapping one another about the children's neck."*

"Dr. Kirton saw a fellow presently removed from a paroxysm of the falling sickness, by cutting off some of his hair, and putting it into his hand."†

In father Jerom Merolla de Sorrento's 'Voyage to Congo,'‡ he mentions the foot of the elk as a certain remedy against epilepsy. The way to find out the foot in which this virtue lies, he says, is to "knock the beast down, when he will immediately lift up that leg which is most efficacious to scratch his ear. Then you must be ready with a sharp scymitar to lop off the medicinal limb, and you shall find an infallible remedy against the falling sickness treasured up in his claws."

Among the Indians and Norwegians and the other northern nations, the hoof of the elk is regarded as a sovereign cure for the epilepsy.

* Blochwick, p. 54.
† Skippon's Account of a Journey in the Low Countries. See Churchill's Collection, vol. vi, p. 656.
‡ Churchill, vol. i., p. 536.

CHARMS.

The person afflicted must apply it to his heart, hold it in his left hand, and rub his ear with it.

Rings composed of different substances have been commonly employed for superstitious purposes. Thus, in Berkshire, Brand* acquaints us that a ring made from a piece of silver collected at the communion, is a cure for convulsions and fits of every kind. If collected on Easter Sunday, its efficacy is greatly increased. Silver is not necessary in Devonshire; in that county they prefer a ring made of three nails or screws that have been used to fasten a coffin, and that have been dug out of the churchyard. In the 'Gentleman's Magazine' for 1794, we are told that a silver ring will cure fits, which is made of five sixpences, collected from five different bachelors, to be conveyed by the hand of a bachelor to a smith that is a bachelor. None of the persons who gave the sixpences are to know for what purpose, or to whom they gave them.

The 'London Medical and Physical Journal' for 1815, notices a charm successfully employed in the cure of epilepsy, after the failure of various medical means. It consisted of a silver ring contributed by twelve young women, and was constantly worn on one of the patient's fingers.

Lupton† says "a piece of a child's navel-string borne in a ring is good against the falling sickness, the pains of the head, and the collick."

Hysteria. Monardes mentions a stone to re-

---

* Popular Antiquities, vol. ii., p. 598.
† Book of Notable Things, p. 92.

lieve hysterical affections: "Cum uteri suffocationem imminentem præsentiunt, adhibito lipide levantur, et si eum perpetuo gestant (hysterici) nunquam simili morbo corripiuntur, exempla hujusmodi faciunt, ut his rebus fidem adhibeam."*

Chorea Sancti Viti. There are many charms against this disease, but none so effectual as an application to the saint. In the translation of Naogeorgus, Barnabe Googe says:

"The nexte is VITUS sodde in oyle, before whose ymage faire
  Both men and women bringing hennes for offring doe repaire:
  The cause whereof I doe not know, I thinke, for some disease
  Which he is thought to drive away from such as him doe please." (Fol. 54 b.)

Madness. Borlase notices† a very singular method of curing madness, mentioned by Carew, in the parish of Altarnum — " to place the disordered in mind on the brink of a square pool, filled with water from St. Nun's well. The patient, having no intimation of what was intended, was, by a sudden blow on the breast, tumbled into the pool, where he was tossed up and down by some persons of superior strength till, being quite debilitated, his fury forsook

---

* [When hysterical persons feel an attack coming on, they may be relieved by a stone, which will prevent, if constantly worn about the person, any subsequent attack. From my knowledge of cases of this kind, I attach credit to this amulet.]

† Natural History of Cornwall, p. 302.

him; he was then carried to church, and certain masses were sung over him. The Cornish call this immersion *boossenning;* from bauzi or bidhyzi in the Cornu-British and Armoric, signifying to dip or drown." Sir Walter Scott notices a practice in Perthshire, where several wells and springs are dedicated to St. Fillan, and are places of pilgrimage and offerings, even among the Protestants:

> " Thence to Saint Fillan's blessed well,
> Whose spring can frenzied dreams dispel,
> And the crazed brain restore."
>
> (*Marmion*, p. 52.)

These wells, the poet tells us, " are held powerful in cases of madness; and, in cases of very late occurrence, lunatics have been left all night bound to the holy stone, in confidence that the saint would come and unloose them before morning." Casting mad people into the sea, or immersing them in water until nigh drowned, have been recommended by high medical authorities as a means of cure. Boerhaave has an aphorism (1123) to this effect: " Præcipitatio in mare, submersio in eo continuata quamdiu ferre potest princeps remedium est."

Palsy, Sciatica, and Lameness. Paracelsus[*] had a ring made of a variety of metallic substances, which he called electrum. He says that rings composed of this metal would prevent the wearers from having either the cramp, palsy,

---

[*] In Archidox. Magic. lib.

apoplexy, epilepsy, or any pain. If the ring be put on during an epileptic fit it would immediately assuage the disease and terminate the fit.

Sleeping on stones, on a particular night, is a method of curing lameness practised in Cornwall.*

The 'Exmoor Scolding' acquaints us that the disease called sciatica is known in the neighbourhood of Exmoor, in Devonshire, by the appellation of 'boneshave;' and that the inhabitants, when affected with this complaint, resort to the use of a charm to be relieved. The patient, it is said, must lie upon his back, on the bank of the river or brook of water, with a straight staff by his side, between him and the water, and must have the following words repeated over him:

> "Boneshave right,
> Boneshave straight,
> As the water runs by the stave,
> Good for boneshave."

Headache. "A halter wherewith any one has been hanged, if tied about the head, will cure the headache. Moss growing upon a human skull, if dried and powdered, and taken as snuff, is no less efficacious."†

Toothache. A nail driven into an oak tree is reported to be a cure for this pain.

Plague. Pestilential diseases have always been regarded as punishments inflicted on man-

---

* Borlase, p. 138. † Grose.

kind for offences and wickedness; and it is not astonishing, therefore, to find that amulets and charms have been prodigally used to avert them. Astrologers attributed the plague to a conjunction of Saturn and Jupiter in Sagittarius, on the 10th of October, or to a conjunction of Saturn and Mars in the same constellation, on the 12th of November. Burton makes the most generous melancholy, as that of Augustus, to come from the conjunction of Saturn and Jupiter in Libra; the bad, as that of Cataline, from the meeting of Saturn and the moon in Scorpio.*—Pouqueville, in his 'Travels in the Morea,' gives an interesting account of the plague as it appeared at Constantinople. The obscurity of its nature and the ravages of its attacks have not unnaturally given rise to a belief in its being an emanation of the celestial vengeance. The natives, we are told, personified it thus: " The evil spirit, or cacodaimon, has been seen to glide along their roofs. No one dares to doubt the assertion. He is a decrepit object, covered with funeral shreds, and has been heard to call by their names those whom he wished to cut off from the number of the living. Nocturnal music and murmuring voices have been heard in the air in the darkest nights, and phantoms have been seen moving in solitary places near the cemeteries. Strange dogs have howled in a dismal manner, and their voices have been terrifically re-echoed along the deserted streets. Thus observed to me an inhabitant of Naupli:

* See Melancthon Lib. de Anima, cap. de Humorib.

'You must take care not to answer if you hear yourself called in the night; you will sometimes be attracted by symphonies — do not listen to them, but cover yourself over in the bed, for it is the decrepit demon — that is, the plague — which knocks at your door."

Mr. Jackson, consul at Mogodor, in his 'Travels in Africa,' gives us an account of the plague which depopulated West Barbary in 1799–1800, and says that the Mohammedans, who are predestinarians and believe in the existence of spirits, devils, &c., regard the plague as a good or blessing sent from God to clear the world of a superfluous population; that no medicine or precaution can cure or prevent it; that every one who is to be a victim to it is (*mktube*) recorded in the book of fate; that there are certain genii who preside over the fate of men, and who sometimes discover themselves in various forms, having often legs similar to those of fowls; that these genii are armed with arrows; that when a person is attacked by the plague, which is called in Arabic *l'amer*, or the destiny or decree, he is shot by one of these genii, and the sensation of the invisible wound is similar to that from a musket-ball; hence the universal application of *M'drob* to a person afflicted with the plague, *i. e.*, he is shot, and if he die *ufah ameruh*, his destiny is completed or terminated — in this world. Mr. Jackson says he scarcely ever yet saw the Mooselmin who did not affirm that he had, at some time of his life, seen these genii, and they often, they say, appear in rivers.

Fear, he observes, had an extraordinary effect

in disposing the body to receive the infection; and those who were subject thereto invariably caught the malady, which was for the most part fatal.

During the severe visitation of the plague in London amulets composed of arsenic were very commonly worn in the region of the heart, upon the principle that one poison would drive out or prevent the entry of another. Large quantities of arsenic were imported into London for this purpose. Dr. Henry wrote against them as " dangerous and hurtful, if not pernitious, to those who weare them."*

Quills of quicksilver were commonly worn about the neck as a preservative against the plague. The powder of toad was employed in a similar way. Pope Adrian is reported never to have been without it. The ingredients forming his amulet were dried toad, arsenic, tormentil, pearl, coral, hyacinth, smarag, and tragacanth. Among the Harleian MSS. is a letter from Lord Chancellor Hatton to Sir Thomas Smith, written at the time of an alarming epidemic. He writes thus: " I am likewise bold to recommend my most humble duty to our dear mistress (Queen Elizabeth) by this LETTER and RING, which hath the virtue to expell infectious airs, and is *to be worn betwixt the sweet duggs*, the chaste nest of pure constancy. I trust, sir, when the virtue is known, it shall not be refused for the value."

Fevers. Brandt† has given a charm for fever,

---

* Preservatives against the Pestilence. Lond. 1625, 4to.
† Popular Antiquities, vol. ii., p. 580.

from a MS., in his possession: "Wryte thys wordys on a lorell lef: + ysmael + ysmael + adjuro vos per angelum ut soporetur iste homo N. and ley thys lef under hys head that he wete not thereof, and let hym ete letuse oft, and drynke ip'e seed smal grounden in a morter, and temper yt with ale."

"The fever," says Werenfels, "he will not drive away by medicines, but, what is a more certain remedy, having pared his nails and tied them to a crayfish, he will turn his back, and as Deucalion did the stones from which a new progeny of men arose, throw them behind him into the next river."

Ague. This fever, of a periodical character, has offered perhaps more opportunities for the employment of charms than any other malady; and there are many cases of cure on record affected by fright or other sudden emotion. All the "horribles" have been pressed into this service; but it will be sufficient for our present purpose to enumerate only a few. Boyle relates the case of a gentleman who entertained great fear of rats. He laboured under an obstinate ague, and was accidentally confined in a room where there was one of those animals, which jumped upon him, and by the fright occasioned by it the ague disappeared. The chain of morbid action which prevailed in the system was broken, and nature then effected the recovery. The chips of a gallows put into a bag and worn round the neck has also been said to have cured ague. Mr. Brand reports to the same effect, and also records[*] that in the Life

Popular Antiquities, vol. ii., p. 583.

of Nicholas Mooney, a notorious highwayman, executed with others at Bristol, in 1752, it is said, that " after the cart drew away, the hangman very deservedly had his head broke for attempting to pull off Mooney's shoes; and a fellow had like to have been killed in mounting the gallows to take away the ropes that were left after the malefactors were cut down. A young woman came fifteen miles for the sake of the rope from Mooney's neck, which was given to her, it being by many apprehended that the halter of an executed person will charm away the ague and perform many other cures."

Elias Ashmole, in his Diary, April 11, 1681, has entered, "I took early in the morning a good dose of elixir, and hung three spiders about my neck, and drove my ague away. Deo Gratias!"

Spiders and their webs have often been recommended for the cure of this malady. Burton gives the following :† " Being in the country in the vacation time, not many years since, at Lindly, in Leicestershire, my father's house, I first observed this amulet of a spider in a nut-shell, wrapped in silk, &c., so applied for an ague by my mother. Whom, although I knew to have excellent skill in chirurgery, sore eyes, aches, &c., and such experimental medicines, as all the country where she dwelt can witness, to have done many famous and good cures upon divers poor folks that were otherwise destitute of help; yet among all other experiments, this methought

* Anatomy of Melancholy, p. 245.

was most absurd and ridiculous. I could see no warrant for it. Quid aranea cum Febre? For what antipathy? till at length rambling amongst authors (as I often do), I found this very medicine in Dioscorides, approved by Matthiolus, repeated by Aldrovandus, cap. de Aranea, lib. de Insectis, I began to have a better opinion of it, and to give more credit to amulets, when I saw it in some parties answer to experience."

Other less offensive means have been employed with the same intent. Thus the Hon. Robert Boyle says* he was cured of a violent quotidian ague, after having in vain resorted to medical aid, by applying to his wrists a mixture of two handfuls of bay salt, the same quantity of fresh English hops, and a quarter of a pound of blue currants, very diligently beaten into a brittle mass, without the addition of anything moist, and so spread upon linen and applied to his wrists. He endeavours to account for this cure by imagining that some of the subtle corpuscles insinuate themselves through the pores of the skin and thus enter the circulation. The wristbands employed in the cure of ague were called Pericarpia. Millefolium or yarrow, worn in a little bag on the pit of the stomach, is also reported to have cured ague.

In Skippon's account of a 'Journey through the Low Countries,' &c., he makes mention of the lectures of Ferrarius and his narrative of the cure of the ague of a Spanish lieutenant, by

---

* Usefulness of Nat. Philosophy, vol. ii., (Works,) ed. Lond. 1772, p. 157.

writing the words FEBRA FUGE, and cutting off a letter from the paper every day, and he observed the distemper to abate accordingly; when he cut the letter F last of all the ague left him. In the same year, he says, fifty more were reported to be cured in the same manner.

Another charm for ague was directed to be said up the chimney, by the eldest female of the family, on St. Agnus Eve. It ran thus:

"Tremble and go!
　First day shiver and burn:
Tremble and quake!
　Second day shiver and learn:
Tremble and die!
　Third day never return."

The possibility of transplanting or transferring the disease was once commonly entertained. Mr. Douce, in some MS. notes transmitted to Mr. Brand, says, "it is usual with many persons about Exeter, who are affected with ague, to visit at dead of night the nearest cross-road five different times, and there bury a new-laid egg. The visit is paid about an hour before the cold fit is expected; and they are persuaded that with the egg they shall bury the ague. If the experiment fail, (and the agitation it occasions may often render it successful,) they attribute it to some unlucky accident that may have befallen them on the way. In the execution of this matter they observe the strictest silence, taking care not to speak to any one whom they may happen to meet." By breaking a salted cake of bran and giving it to a dog, when the fit comes on, the malady has been supposed to be transferred from the patient to the animal.

Serenus Samonicus affords us a classical remedy for a quartan ague, by placing the fourth book of Homer's Iliad under the patient's head. An enumeration of these follies might be extended to a great length; but I shall close this part of my subject by a narrative of considerable interest, relating to Sir John Holt, Lord Chief Justice of the Court of King's Bench, 1709, who, it is said, was extremely wild in his youth, and being once engaged with some of his rakish friends in a trip into the country, in which they had spent all their money, it was agreed they should try their fortune separately. Holt arrived at an inn at the end of a straggling village, ordered his horse to be taken care of, bespoke a supper and a bed. He then strolled into the kitchen, where he observed a little girl of thirteen shivering with an ague. Upon making inquiry respecting her, the landlady told him that she was her only child, and had been ill nearly a year, notwithstanding all the assistance she could procure for her from physic. He gravely shook his head at the doctors, bade her be under no further concern, for that her daughter should never have another fit. He then wrote a few unintelligible words in a court hand on a scrap of parchment, which had been the direction affixed to a hamper, and rolling it up, directed that it should be bound upon the girl's wrist and there allowed to remain until she was well. The ague returned no more; and Holt, having remained in the house a week,

CHARMS. 97

called for his bill. "God bless you, Sir," said the old woman, "you're nothing in my debt, I'm sure. I wish, on the contrary, that I was able to pay you for the cure which you have made of my daughter. Oh! if I had had the happiness to see you ten months ago, it would have saved me forty pounds." With pretended reluctance he accepted his accommodation as a recompense, and rode away. Many years elapsed, Holt advanced in his profession of the law, and went a circuit, as one of the judges of the Court of King's Bench, into the same county, where, among other criminals brought before him, was an old woman under a charge of witchcraft. To support this accusation, several witnesses swore that the prisoner had a spell with which she could either cure such cattle as were sick or destroy those that were well, and that in the use of this spell she had been lately detected, and that it was now ready to be produced in court. Upon this statement the judge desired it might be handed up to him. It was a dirty ball, wrapped round with several rags, and bound with packthread. These coverings he carefully removed, and beneath them found a piece of parchment, which he immediately recognized as his own youthful fabrication. For a few moments he remained silent — at length, recollecting himself, he addressed the jury to the following effect: "Gentlemen, I must now relate a particular of my life, which very ill suits my present character and the station in which I sit; but to conceal it would be to aggravate the folly for which I ought to atone, to endanger innocence, and to countenance superstition. This bauble, which you suppose to have the power of life and death, is a senseless scroll which I wrote with my own hand and gave to this woman, whom for no other reason you accuse as a witch." He then related the particulars of the transaction, with such an effect upon the minds of the people, that his old landlady was the last person tried for witchcraft in that country.

Hectic Fever and Consumption. Many physical charms were in use in different parts of Scotland. In the province of Moray, the Rev. Mr. Shaw tells us, in his history of that place, that in hectic and consumptive diseases, the inhabitants pare the nails of the fingers and toes of the patient, put them into a rag cut from his clothes, then wave their hand with the rag thrice round his head, crying, *Deas soil;* after which they bury the rag in some unknown place. This is a practice similar to that recorded by Pliny, as practised by the magicians and Druids of his time.

In the Highlands of Scotland is an affection of the chest, known by the appellation of Glacach or Macdonald's disease, because there are tribes of that name who are considered to have the power, by the use of a certain set of words, of removing the complaint. No fee of any kind is to be given.

Hooping-cough. It is a common superstition in Devonshire, Cornwall, and some other parts of England, to inquire of any one riding on a pyeball horse of a remedy for the hooping-cough, and whatever may be named is regarded as an infallible specific.

Gout. The attacks of this disease are often periodical, and they have been subjected to the influence of charms. Alexander of Tralles, a medical writer of celebrity, has given the following as an esteemed one in his time: "Remedium a Podagrâ præservans in laminam auream, lunâ desinente, quæ sequuntur inscribito, et nervis gruis involvito: deinde simili canaliculo ipsam includito, gestatoque ad talos. Meu, treu, mor, phor, teux, za, zor, phe, lou, chri, ge, ze, on. Quemadmodum sol in hisce remediis firmatur, et quotidie renovatur, ita hoc figmentum confirmatur quemadmodum prius. Jam, jam, cito, cito, ecce enim magnum nomen dico in quo conquiescentia firmantur. Jaz, Azyph, Zyon, threux, bayn, choog. Firmate hoc figmentum ut erat primum. Jam, jam, cito, cito. Ad Podagram, quæ nondum contraxit nodos, admirabile et probatum."*

Scrofula. For this disease many charms have been employed, but no remedy has been so highly esteemed as the royal touch, of which a particular history is given in another part of this volume. The hand of the sovereign, however, was by some deemed not more efficacious than that of a murderer or of a virgin; for in Scot's 'Discovery of Witchcraft' it is stated, "To heal

* [A remedy for the gout. Write, on a golden plate at the wane of the moon, what follows, rolling round it the sinews of a crane. Put it in a little bag, and wear it near the ankles. The words are meu, treu, &c.]

† Lib. xi., cap. 1.

the king or queen's evil, or any other soreness of the throat, first touch the place with the hand of one that died an untimely death, otherwise let a virgin, fasting, lay her hand on the sore, and say, 'Apollo denyeth that the heat of the plague can increase where a naked virgin quencheth it;' and spit three times upon it." To dispel tumours, particularly of a scrofulous nature, the stroking nine times with the hand of a dead man, and particularly of one who has suffered a violent death as the penalty of his crimes, especially if it be for murder, has been a common practice, and, if not followed at the present day, was certainly a few years since, it being no unfrequent thing to observe on the scaffold numbers of persons submitting to this disgusting foolery, under the exercise of the executioner and his assistants.

"Squire Morley, of Essex, used to say a prayer, which he hoped would do no harm when he hung a bit of vervain-root from a scrofulous person's neck. My aunt Freeman had a very high opinion of a baked toad, in a silk bag, hung round the neck."*

Rickets. This is a modification of scrofula, and children thus affected have been drawn through a cleft tree, which was afterwards bound up, and as it united, the disease disappeared or the child gained strength. Grose says, that if a tree of any kind is split, and weak, rickety, or ruptured children drawn through it and the tree afterwards bound up, as the tree

---

* Brand's Popular Antiquities, vol. ii., p. 598.

heals and grows together, so will the children acquire strength. Sir John Cullum saw the operation performed, and states that the ash tree was selected as the most preferable for the purpose. It was split longitudinally about five feet: the fissure was kept open by the gardener, whilst the friend of the child, having first stripped him naked, passed him thrice through it, almost head foremost. This accomplished, the tree was bound up with packthread, and as he bark healed, so it was said the child would ecover. One of the cases was of rickets, the ther a rupture. The ash tree has been very enerally preferred for superstitious practices. White, in his well-known 'Natural History of Selborne,' has noticed this particularly. Not only trees, but stones, were similarly used. To creep through a perforated stone was a Druidical ceremony; and in the parish of Marden there is, or was, a stone with a hole in it fourteen inches in diameter, through which children were drawn for the rickets.

Sore Eyes. This is another scrofulous disorder. Willielmus de Montibus, chancellor of the mother church of Lincoln, has given a blessing and a ceremonial in which it is to be conferred, for the cure of sore eyes.* Cotta† relates "a merrie historie of an approved famous spell for sore eyes. By many honest testimonies it was a long time worne as a jewell about

---

* See Beckett's Collection of Records, No. iv.

† Short Discoverie of the Dangers of ignorant Practisers of Physicke, p. 49.

many necks, written in paper and inclosed in silke, never failing to do sovereigne good when all other helpes were helplesse. No sight might dare to reade or open. At length a curious mind, while the patient slept, by stealth ripped open the mystical cover, and found the powerful characters Latin: 'Diabolus effodiat tibi oculos, impleat foramina stercoribus.'"

Marasmus. Mr. Boyle tells the case of a physician whom he consulted, and whose wan looks — probably as bad as those of the meagre apothecary of Shakespeare in 'Romeo and Juliet' — betokened a marasmus, and who was induced, failing in other means, to employ a sympathetic mode of treatment. He took an egg and boiled it hard in his own warm urine; he then with a bodkin perforated the shell in many places, and buried it in an ant-hill, where it was kept to be devoured by the emmets; and as they wasted the egg, he found his distemper to abate and his strength to increase, insomuch that his disease left him.

Calculus. For the cure of stone, Boyle tells us that the Lapis nephriticus — a species of jasper — was frequently bound at the wrists, but chiefly on that of the left hand. Anselmus Boetius de Boot, Monardes, Untzerus, and Johannes de Laet have borne evidence to its efficacy.*

Cholera. The Lapis porcinus, according to

---

* Boot de Lapid. et Gem., lib. ii., cap. 11. Monardes de Simplic. Ind. Hist., 20. Untzerus de Nephrit., lib. i., cap. 24. Boyle's Usefulness of Natural Philosophy (Works), vol. ii., cap. 10, p. 156.

Bontius, is declared to be good for the cholera, but it must not be given to pregnant women. It was sufficient for the females of Malaica to hold the stone in their hands to produce the catamenia, if obstruction existed.

During the prevalence of cholera a few years since, it was common in many parts of Austria, Germany, and Italy, to wear an amulet at the pit of the stomach, in contact with the skin. I have one of these, sent from Hungary; it consists merely of a circular piece of copper, two inches and a half in diameter, and is without characters. In Naples, I learn, they were very generally worn.

Jaundice. Seven or nine — it must be an odd number — cakes made of the newly emitted and warm urine of the patient with the ashes of ash wood, and buried for some days in a dunghill, will, according to Paracelsus, cure the yellow jaundice. This is called a cure by transplantation.

In the Journal of Dr. Edward Browne, transmitted to his father, Sir Thomas Browne, we read of "a magical cure for the jaundice: Burne wood under a leaden vessel filled with water; take the ashes of that wood, and boyle it with the patient's urine; then lay nine long heaps of the boyld ashes upon a board in a ranke, and upon every heap lay nine spears of crocus: it hath greater effects than is credible to any one that shall barely read this receipt without experiencing."*

---

* Works, vol. i., p. 48.

A letter from Mr. Hann to the Hon. Robert Boyle gives some instances of transplantation: The cure of jaundice by the burying in a dunghill a cake made of ashes and the patient's urine. Ague in a boy cured by a cake made of barley-meal and his urine, and given to a dog to eat — the dog had a shaking fit, and the boy was cured. Boys cured of warts by taking an elder-stick and cutting as many notches in it as there were warts, then rubbing it upon the warts and burying it in a dunghill.* Salmuth also relates a case of cure by transplantation: "The patient had a most violent pain of the arm, and they beat up red corals with oaken leaves, and having kept them on the part affected till suppuration, they did in the morning put this mixture into a hole bored with an augur in the root of an oak, respecting the east, and stop up this hole with a peg made of the same tree; from thenceforth the pain did altogether cease, and when they took out the amulet immediately the torments returned sharper than before."†

Worms. Charms were often employed for the cure of worms, accompanied with a form of prayer. Brand quotes a MS. which contained an exorcism against all kinds of worms which infest the body: it was to be repeated three mornings as a certain remedy.

Bites of Venomous Animals. Serpents' bites were said to be healed by a company of people called sauveurs, who had a mark of St. Catha-

---

* Vol. vi., p. 168.

† See on this subject, Bartholinus de Transplantatione Morborum, Hafniæ, 1673, 12mo.

rine's wheel upon their palate. Snake-stones were originally brought from Java, and supposed by their absorbent power to have the quality of extracting the poison inserted, by being simply placed over the bitten part. Charms are common in Aleppo against scorpions, serpents, bugs, and other vermin. Russell* mentions one in particular against musquitoes. It consists of a little slip of paper, on which is inscribed certain unintelligible characters, and this is pasted upon the lintel of a door, or over the windows. The power of distributing these charms has descended hereditarily in one family, and on a certain day in the year they are given gratis. In 'Navarette's Account of the Phillipine Islands'† he alludes to the abundance of scorpions, and was told that the best remedy against them was, when going to bed, to make a commemoration of St. George. This devotion, he says, he continued many years, and the saint failed not to deliver him from the tormentors. The bed was also rubbed with garlic, which doubtless was by far the most efficacious part of the remedy. Pierius mentions the following against the sting of the scorpion: "The patient is to sit on an ass, with his face to the tail of the animal, by which the pain will be transmitted from the man to the beast." Pontanus records a charm used by the people of Apulia for the bite of the tarantula, and which was found equally efficacious against the bite of a mad dog. This was,

* Hist. of Aleppo, p. 103.
† Churchill's Collection of Voyages, vol. i., p. 212.

to go *nine* times round the town on the Sabbath, calling upon and imploring the assistance of the saint. On the *third* night — the prayers being heard and granted, and the disease restored — the madness was removed. The charm runs thus:

> "Alme vithe pellicane,
> Oram qui tenes Apulam,
> Littusque polyganicum,
> Qui Morsus rabidos levas,
> Irasque canum mitigas:
> Tu, Sancte, Rabiem asperam,
> Rictusque canis luridos,
> Tu sævam prohibe luem.
> I procul hinc Rabies,
> Procul hinc furor omnis abesto."*

Erysipelas. Bollandus gives an account of many miracles wrought by the intercession of St. Anthony, particularly in the distemper called *Sacred Fire*, which since his time has been called *St. Anthony's Fire*, it having miraculously ceased through his patronage when raging violently in many parts of Europe in the eleventh century. Blochwick mentions an amulet against erysipelas. It is to be made of the "Elder on which the sun never shined. If the piece betwixt the two knots be hung about the patient's neck, it is much commended. Some cut it in little pieces, and sew it in a knot

---

* [Thou who presidest over the Apulian shores,
Thou who curest the bites of mad dogs,
Thou, O Sacred One, ward off this cruel plague,
This dismal gnawing of dogs.
Get thee far hence, O madness, O fury.]

CHARMS.

in a piece of a man's shirt, which seems superstitious."

Herpes. Turner* notices a prevalent charm among old women for the shingles: the blood of a black cat, taken from the cat's tail and smeared on the part affected. In the only case, however, in which he saw this superstition practised, it caused considerable mischief.

Burns. In Pepys's Diary† there is "A charme for a burning :"

> "There came three angels out of the east;
> The one brought fire, the other brought frost—
> Out fire; in frost:
> In the name of the Father, and Son, and Holy Ghost.
> Amen."

Thorns. The same authority records "A charme for a thorne :"

> "Jesus, that was of a Virgin born,
>   Was pricked both with nail and thorn;
>   It neither wealed, nor belled, rankled nor boned;
>   In the name of Jesus no more shall this."

Or, thus:

> "Christ was of a Virgin born,
>   And he was pricked with a thorn;
>   And it did neither bell, nor swell;
>   And I trust in Jesus this never will."

Reginald Scott‡ gives a charm used in the

---

* Diseases of the Skin, p. 82.
† Vol. i., p. 323.
‡ Discovery of Witchcraft, p. 137.

Romish Church upon St. Blaze's day, that will fetch a thorn out of any place of one's body, a bone out of the throat, &c., to wit: "Call upon God, and remember St. Blaze."

Warts. For the charming of warts many means have been devised; several of these are ridiculous and disgusting. Grose gives, for the removal of these excrescences, direction to "steal a piece of beef from a butcher's shop, and rub your wart with it, then throw it down the necessary-house, or bury it, and as the beef rots, your warts will decay." Sir Thomas Browne says, "for warts we rub our hands before the moon, and commit any maculated part to the touch of the dead."

Sir Kenelm Digby says,[*] "One would think it were a folly that one should offer to wash his hands in a well-polished silver basin, wherein there is not a drop of water, yet this may be done by the reflection of the moonbeams only, which will afford it a competent humidity to do it; but they who have tried it, have found their hands, after they are wiped, to be much moister than usually; but this is an infallible way to take away warts from the hands, if it be often used."

Small-pox. This is a disease of great antiquity. It was known at a very early period in China and in India; and there is a Chinese[†] as well as an Indian goddess, who is conceived to have a superintending power over the disease. The Hindoo goddess has been particularly described

---

[*] Discourse on the Power of Sympathy.
[†] See Hist. of China, by Père de Halde, vol. iv.

by Mr. Moore, from an original drawing, which is exceedingly curious.* Inoculation was practised at a very early period in Hindostan,† and during the ceremony prayers appointed in the Attharva Veda, were solemnly recited to propitiate the goddess. A small present was also made to the Bramin officiating, who never failed to lay an injunction on the family; also to make a thanksgiving offering to the goddess upon their recovery from the disease. Mr. Moore has quoted an exorcism from a MS. in the Harleian Collection,‡ which reads thus: "In nomine Patris, et Filii, et Spiritus Sancti, amen. + in adjutorium sit Salvator noster + dominus celi .... audi preces famulorum famularumque tuarum Domine Jhesu Chrispte.... adque peto Angelorum milia aut (ut) me + sol-

---

* "The Small-pox goddess stands with two uplifted crooked daggers, threatening to strike on the right and left. Before her are a band of the executers of her vengeance. Two of them wear red grinning masks, carry black shields, and brandish naked scymitars. White lines, like rays, issue from the bodies of the others, to indicate infection. On the right, there is a group of men with spotted bodies, inflicted with the malady: bells are hung at their cinctures, and a few of them wave in their hands black feathers. They are preceded by musicians with drums, who are supplicating the pity of the furious deity. Behind the goddess, on the right, there advances a bevy of smiling young women, who are carrying gracefully on their heads baskets with thanksgiving-offerings, in gratitude for their lives and their beauty having been spared. There is, besides, a little boy with a bell at his 'girdle, who seems to be conveying something from the right arm of the goddess. This action may possibly be emblematic of inoculation." (History of the Small-pox, p. 33.)

† Chais Essai Apolog., &c., p. 220.

‡ Number 585, p. 202.

vent ac defendant doloris igniculo et potestate Variola, ac protegat mortis a periculo; tuas Jhesu Chrispte aures tuas nobis inclina."* The same MS. gives a prayer addressed to St. Nicaise for the consecration of an amulet against the disease. It is in barbarous Latin, but may be rendered thus: "In the name of our Lord Jesus Christ, may the Lord protect these persons, and may the work of these virgins ward off the small-pox. St. Nicaise had the small-pox, and he asked the Lord (to preserve) whoever carried his name inscribed: O, St. Nicaise! thou illustrious biohop and martyr, pray for me, a sinner, and defend me by thy intercession from this disease. Amen."

Hemorrhage and Hemorrhoids. Precious stones, stones of various composition, verses, disgusting animals, &c., have all been put into requisition for the suppression of hemorrhagy. Garcias ab Orto† makes mention of a stone called alaqueca, found in Balagat, the virtue of which is accounted above all other gems, inasmuch as it is able to stop the flux of blood in any part. Monardes mentions the Lapis sanguinaris, or blood-stone, found in New Spain, of which the Indians believe that if it be applied

---

* [In the name of the Father, the Son, and Holy Spirit, amen .... + may our Saviour be our help + the lord of Heaven ..... hear the prayers of thy servants and handmaidens, Lord Jesus Christ; and I ask for a thousand angels + that they may protect me from the contagion of the small-pox and the danger of death. Incline thy ears to us, Jesus Christ.]

† Lib. ii., cap. 53.

to any recent wound it will immediately check the bleeding; and he says that he has seen persons afflicted with hemorrhoids who wore this stone in rings on their fingers for relief. The jasper, which is blood-red throughout, has been highly celebrated for its power in controlling hemorrhage. Boetius de Boot says* he cured a maid at Prague, who had suffered from a violent hemorrhagy for six years, for which she had often been bled, and various remedies resorted to without effect, by merely hanging a jasper round her neck which effected her cure. Upon leaving off the jasper the hemorrhage would return, and this continued to be the case for some time; at length, however, she was perfectly cured.

Van Helmont affirms that he had a metal, of which, if a ring were made and worn, not only the pain attendant upon hemorrhoids would cease, but that in twenty-four hours, whether internal or external, they would vanish altogether.† Brandt‡ gives "A charme to staunch blood: Jesus that was in Bethleem born, and baptyzed was in the flumen Jordane, as stente the water at hys comyng, so stente the blood of thys man N. thy servvaunt, thorw the virtu of thy holy Name + Jesu + & of thy Cosyn swete Sent Jon. And sey thys charme fyve tymes with fyve Pater Nosters, in the worschep of the fyve woundys." Pepys, in his 'Diary,' gives also the following:

* De Lapid. et Gem., lib. ii., cap. 102.
† Lib. de Febrib., cap. ii.
‡ Popular Antiquities, vol. ii., p. 580.

"FOR STENCHING OF BLOOD.

> Sanguis mane in te,
> Sicut Christus fuit in se;
> Sanguis mane in tuâ venâ,
> Sicut Christus in suâ pœnâ;
> Sanguis mane fixus,
> Sicut Christus quando fuit crucifixus."*

Homer refers to the suppression of bleeding from the wound received by Ulysses, by a charm; and Sir Walter Scott, in the 'Lay of the Last Minstrel,' says:

> "She drew the splinter from the wound,
> And with a CHARM she staunch'd the blood."

Toads, either alive or dried, and laid upon the back of the neck, are often mentioned as a means of stopping a bleeding at the nose. They were formed into a powder, called the Pulvis Æthiopicus, of which the mode of preparation is given in Bates's 'Pharmacopœia.' It was used externally and also given internally in cases of dropsy, small-pox, and other diseases.

Boyle says,† "Having been one summer frequently subject to bleeding at the nose, and reduced to employ several remedies to check that

---

* [Blood remain in Thee,
As Christ was in himself;
Blood remain in thy veins,
As Christ in his pains;
Blood remain fixed,
As Christ was on the crucifix.]

† Essay on Porousness of Animal Bodies, vol. iv. (Works), p. 767.

distemper; that whch I found the most effectual to stanch the blood was some moss of a dead man's skull, (sent for a present out of Ireland, where it is far less rare than in most other countries,) though it did but touch my skin, till the herb was a little warmed by it."

Sterility. The Abbé Mariti* has given a description of the mandrake, the fruit of which, he says, is very exhilarating and a provocative of venery. The application of mandrakes, as remedies for sterility, is professed to have been taken from the history of Jacob and Leah.† The fabulous conceits relating to this plant are well exposed by Sir Thomas Browne, in his 'Pseudodoxia Epidemica.' The fancied resemblance of the root to the shape of the limbs of a man is likely to have caused its employment against barrenness, in accordance with the opinion entertained of an agreement or correspondence of power and form.

Childbirth. The superstitious practices connected with this state are numerous. At the time of an accouchement, charms seem formerly to have been much employed. Bonner, bishop of London in 1554, forbids‡ "a mydwife of his diocese to exercise any witchecrafte, charmes, sorcerye, invocations, or praiers, other than such as be allowable and may stand with the lawes and ordinances of the Catholike Churche."

---

* Travels, vol. ii., p. 195.
† Genesis, chap. xxx.
‡ Injunctions at the Visitation from Sept. 3, 1554, to Oct. 8, 1555.

And in 1559, (1st Eliz.,) an inquiry* was directed to be made "whether you knowe any that doe use charmes, sorcery, enchauntementes, invocations, circles, witchecraftes, southsayinge, or any lyke craftes or imaginacions invented by the devyl, and specially in the tyme of women's travaylle." Strype† tells us that in 1567 the midwives took an oath, *inter alia*, not to "suffer any other bodies' child to be set, brought, or laid before any woman delivered of child in the place of her natural child, so far forth as I can know and understand. Also I will not use any kind of sorcerye or incantation in the time of the travail of any woman."

To promote or facilitate delivery, the Lapis ætites, or eagle-stone, a composition of the oxyde of iron with small portions of silex and alumina, which rattle within upon being shook, have been bound to the arm or to the thigh, the former to prevent abortion, the latter to aid in parturition. "Aquilæ lapis qui in ventre ejus aut in nido inventus fuerit, phylacterium est prægnantibus. Nomen habet Ætites."‡ "Iris helpeth a woman to speedie deliverance, and maketh rainebows to appeare." The sardonyx was laid *inter mammas*, to procure easy birth, and one formerly belonged to the monastery of St. Alban's to be used for this purpose.§ The Chinese re-

---

* Articles to be inquired in the Visitacyon in the fyrst yeare of Queen Eliz., 1559.

† Annals of the Reformation, vol. i., p 537.

‡ Sextus Philosophus Platonicus de Medicina Animalium, &c. Tiguri, 1539, p. 100.

§ Brand's Popular Antiquities, vol. ii., p. 599, note.

commend, with the same intention, a marine insect in the shape of a horse, which is to be held in the hand of the woman in labour, and she will then be delivered of her burthen with the same facility "as a ewe which has gone her full time." Branches of palm were also held in the hand by child-bearing women.*

The men in some countries, when the women are delivered, lie in, keep their bed, and are attended as if really sick.† At Surinam, Fermin says, the man keeps to his *hamac* for six weeks. In Persia, when a woman is about to lie in, the school-masters are requested to give liberty to their boys, and birds confined in cages are permitted to escape. Charlevoix says, that when the women of Maroc perceive labour-pains, the neighbours select five school-boys, and tie four eggs in the four corners of a napkin, with which the boys run singing through the streets.

Child's Caul. In this and some other countries when a child is born with the caul or amnion over its face, it is preserved with great care and regarded as ominous of good fortune to the infant, and also as valuable to any one who may become possessed of it, enabling them to avoid many serious dangers. "Il est né coiffé," is a French proverb applied to lucky people. In Scotland, according to Ruddiman,‡ it is called

---

* Homer in Hymn. Apoll. v. 14.

† See on this subject the works of Biet, Du Tertre, Thevet, Lafitau, Froger, Boulanger, &c. Similar accounts are to be found in the writings of Diodorus Siculus, Apollonius, and Strabo.

‡ Glossary to Douglas's Virgil.

a *haly* or *sely how*, a holy or fortunate cap or hood. A midwife in Scotland is called a howdy or howdy wife. The virtues of the caul are described as various; it renders advocates eloquent, saves the possessor from having his house destroyed by fire, or being himself drowned. It is therefore much in request with seafaring people, and may be seen among the advertisements of our newspapers when to be disposed of at a considerable price.

Cramp. For this affection many charms in verse are extant. The following is from Pepys's 'Diary :'*

> " Cramp, be thou faintless,
> As our Lady was sinless
> When she bare Jesus."

Rings have, however, constituted the principal means for the prevention or cure of cramp. They may be of various kinds; and were frequently composed of iron that had previously formed the hinges of a coffin. Andrew Boorde, who lived in the reign of Henry VIII, speaking of the cramp says, "The kynges majesty hath a great helpe in this matter, in hallowynge crampe rynges, and so given without money or petition." Also " the kynges of Englande doth halowe every yere crampe rynges, ye which rynges worne on ones fynger doth helpe them whych hath the crampe." This ceremonial was practised by previous sovereigns and discontinued by Edward VI. Queen Mary intended to revive it; but does not appear to have

---

* Vol. i., p. 324.

carried her intentions into effect. Hospinian* gives an account of the ceremony, and states that it was performed upon Good Friday, and that it originated from a ring which had been brought to King Edward by some persons from Jerusalem, and one which he himself hath long before given privately to a poor petitioner who asked alms of him for the love he bore to St. John the Evangelist. This ring was preserved with great veneration in Westminster Abbey, and whoever was touched by this relic was said to be cured of the cramp or of the falling sickness.† Burnet acquaints us‡ that Bishop Gardiner was at Rome in 1529, and that he wrote a letter to Ann Boleyn, by which it appears that Henry VIII blessed the cramp rings before as well as after the separation from Rome, and that she sent them as great presents thither. " Mr. Stephens, I send you here cramp rings for you and Mr. Gregory and Mr. Peter, praying you to distribute them as you think best. ANN BOLEYN." Burnet adds, " the use of them had been (it seems) discontinued in King Edward's time, but now, under Queen Mary, it was designed to be revived, and the office for it was written out in a fair manuscript, yet extant," of which Burnet has put a copy in his collection.§

* De Origine Festor. Christianor.
† See also Polydore Virgil, lib. viii.
‡ Hist. of the Reformation, vol. ii., p. 644, ed. 1829.
§ No. 25, vol. ii., part 2, pp. 414–17. The office of consecrating the cramp-rings printed by Burnet is from a MS. in Biblioth. R. Smith, London. Beckett has also given the Form of Prayer in his Collection of Records, No. V. See also Waldron's Literary Museum.

The silence in the writers of that time makes him think it was seldom, if ever, practised.

In the Liber Niger Domus Regis Edw. IV, is inserted, "Item, to the kynge's offerings to the crosse on Good Friday, out from the countyng-house for medycinable rings of gold and silver, delyvered to the jewell house, xxv s."

Incubus. Stones with holes through them were commonly called hag-stones, and were often attached to the key of the stable door to prevent witches riding the horses. One of these suspended at the bed's head was celebrated for the prevention of night-mare. It is mentioned by Burton, Browne, Grose, and several other authors. The superstition is thus noticed in Lluellin's Poems :

"Some the night-mare hath prest
  With that weight on their brest,
    No returnes of their breath can passe,
  But to us the tale is addle,
  We can take off her saddle,
    And turn out the night-mare to grasse." (p. 36.)

ON THE INFLUENCE OF THE MIND UPON THE BODY.

"Medical cannot be separated from moral science, without reciprocal and essential mutilation." REID.

THE various cases now adduced in which talismans, amulets, and charms have been employed, either to avert or to cure different diseases, are, in any explanation that can be offered, to be referred to the influence of the mind over the functions of the body. The occasional cures that have followed their employment can only be attributed to the operation of the imagination, by which it is possible that changes may have been effected in the human body and healthy action induced. The efficiency of charms has been in proportion to the ignorance of the age in which they have been used, and the consequent degree of superstition entertained, at a period when the hallucinations of the imagination were permitted to usurp the place of observation, and the greatest puerilities superseded the employment of reason and experiment. In early times, therefore, the instances are numerous — they are now comparatively rare, and occur only in districts not remarkable for intellectual enlightenment. The force of imagination and the power of fear exercised on the animal economy are admitted by every one, but the limits to which their operations are to be assigned no one can designate. Medical observers constantly meet with extraordinary changes produced upon the body from passions of the mind or sudden emotions. Jaundice has been known to occur almost instantaneously upon a violent fit of anger, or within twenty-four hours of the receipt of bad intelligence or the occurrence of unexpectedly severe losses. The hair which was jet black shall in a few hours lose its colour, be deprived of its natural secretion, and turn gray or white, and this may be either partial or general.

> "For deadly fear can time outgo,
> And blaunch at once the hair."— (*Marmion.*)

Some remarkable instances of this kind are to be found in Schenckius.* One of a noble Spaniard, Don Diego Osorio, who being in love with a young lady of the court, had prevailed with her for a private conference within the gardens of the king; but by the barking of a little dog their privacy was betrayed, the young gentleman seized by the king's guard and imprisoned. It was capital to be found in that place, and therefore he was condemned to die. He was so terrified at hearing this sentence, that one and the same night saw the same person young and old, being turned gray, as in those stricken in years. The gaoler, moved at the sight, related the accident to King Ferdinand

* Observ. Med. Rarior., p. 2.

as a prodigy, who thereupon pardoned him, saying, he had been sufficiently punished for his fault. A nobleman of the Roman court was also detected in an intrigue, cast into prison, and sentenced to be decapitated on the morrow. When brought before the Emperor Cæsar he was so altered by the apprehension of death that his identity was questioned; the comeliness and beauty of his face being vanished, his countenance like a dead man's, his hair and beard turned gray, and in all respects so changed that the emperor caused strict examination of him to be made, and to ascertain whether his hair and beard had not been changed by art; this, however, being satisfactorily proved not to be the case, the emperor, moved to pity, graciously pardoned him. The Hon. Robert Boyle mentions partial cases which occurred during the Irish rebellion. Borelli gives an instance of a French gentleman, who upon being thrown into prison was so powerfully affected by fear, that his hair changed completely to a gray in the course of the night. He was released and the hair recovered its colour.*

The effects of fear upon the body are apparent in many other ways. An approach to the door of a dentist by one labouring under toothache has often been found a sure means of banishing violent pain. Fright has frequently cured ague and other disorders of a periodical character; even fits of the gout have been terminated in the same manner. Paralysed mus-

---

* Cent. i., Obs. 37.

cles, and limbs that were useless, have suddenly been thrown into action, and hemorrhages have as instantaneously been checked. The same causes productive of disease have been found also to effect their cure. Dr. Pfeuffer knew a girl in the vicinity of Wurzburg, who, after being deaf for several years, instantly regained her hearing upon being made acquainted with the sudden death of her father. Every one has heard of the treatment proposed by the celebrated Boerhaave, to restrain imitative epilepsy by branding the next who should be affected with a hot iron. Dr. Scott relates a case in which a threat to apply a red-hot iron to the feet of a boy who had been frequently attacked with epilepsy upwards of a year, was perfectly successful in preventing the recurrence of the disease.

A variety of conjectures might be offered to account for many of these phenomena, but none would be perfectly satisfactory to the minute and philosophical inquirer. Too much attention, however, cannot be paid to that mysterious union which exists between mind and body. The ancients were well convinced of this, though they effected little towards turning their opinion to advantage. Plato says, " The office of the physician extends equally to the purification of mind and body; to neglect the one is to expose the other to evident peril. It is not only the body that by its sound constitution strengthens the soul, but the well-regulated soul by its authoritative power maintains the body in perfect health." The mind without the body, nor the body without the mind, cannot be well. "Non sine animo corpus, nec sine corpore animus bene valere potest."

Sir Alexander Crichton, in his admirable work on 'Mental Derangement,' in which he has no less powerfully than philosophically delineated the several passions and their varied operations, observes, that "the passions are to be considered, in a medical point of view, as a part of our constitution, which is to be examined with the eye of a natural historian, and the spirit and impartiality of a philosopher." At a meeting (1834) of the British Association for the Advancement of Science, Dr. Abercrombie drew the attention of the medical section to the importance of the study of mental philosophy. He urged the propriety of treating it as a branch of physiology, and recommended the cultivation of it on strict philosophical principles as a science of observation, and as likely to yield laws, principles, or universal facts, which might be ascertained with the same precision as the laws of physical science. He, however, abjured all speculations respecting the nature and essence of mind, and contended for the necessity of confining these researches to a simple and careful study of its operations. The purposes to which this study should be applied, in the opinion of this learned physician and most excellent man, were the education of the young and the cultivation of a sound mental discipline at any period of life — the intellectual and moral treatment of insanity — the prevention of this disease in individuals in whom there exists the hereditary predisposition to it — and the study of mental science as the basis of a philosophical logic.

Too little attention is paid by physicians in general to the influence of the mind or the operations of the passions in the production and in the removal of disease. We know, it is true, that some of the passions excite whilst others depress; and we see how quickly and how often permanently changes are produced in the offices of different parts of the body. Whilst anger, on the one hand, accelerates the progress of the blood, hurrying on the circulation with fearful impetuosity, to the destruction of either the brain or the organs contained within the chest; grief, on the other, depresses the action of the heart, and causes serious accumulations in the larger vessels and in the lungs. Grief has not inaptly been styled "a heavy executioner; nothing more crucifies the soul, nor overthrows the health of the body than sorrow." The Psalmist beautifully expresses it: "My soul melteth away for very heaviness." Shakspeare's picture is not more true morally than physically, when he makes Macbeth to ask the physician:

> "Canst thou minister to a mind diseas'd,
> Pluck from the memory a rooted sorrow,
> Raze out the written troubles of the brain,
> And with some sweet oblivious antidote
> Cleanse the stuff'd bosom of that perilous stuff
> Which weighs upon the heart?"*

---

* Mr. Collier's excellent edition. Steevens substituted the word foul for stuff'd, which is in the old copies. Stuffed, however, is the right word, and justly expresses the sensation

Violent grief may be speedy and fatal in its effects, but that which is slow and continued is most inimical to health. It undermines the strongest and best of constitutions, and is the cause of a long catalogue of diseases. The energy of the nervous system is weakened, the functions are carried on in a slow and an unequal manner, so that in these cases the body and soul may literally be said "reciprocally to prey on each other."

"'Tis painful thinking that corrodes our clay."
(ARMSTRONG.)

From the operation of anger or of grief, either in excess or under a modified condition, various disorders may arise; and to the influence of the passions generally, therefore, in health as well as in disease, should the attention of the medical practitioner be directed. It has been well said by Dr. Reid, that he who in the study or the treatment of the human machinery, overlooks the intellectual part of it, cannot but entertain very incorrect notions of its nature, and fall into gross and sometimes fatal blunders in the means which he adopts for its regulation or repair. Intellect is not omnipotent; but its actual power over the organized matter to which it is attached is much greater than is usually imagined. The

experienced; there is, however, an unpleasant effect produced by the word stuff occurring so soon after it, and Mr. C. observes that the error, if there be any, lies in the last word of the line; probably there may have been some error by the printer.

anatomy of the mind, therefore, should be learnt, as well as that of the body; the study of its constitution in general, and its peculiarities, or what may be technically called its idiosyncrasies, in any individual case, ought to be regarded as one of the most essential branches of a medical education.

The power of the mind exerted over the body has been rendered conspicuous by many remarkable cases on record:

> "Men may die of imagination,
> So depe may impression be take."
> (CHAUCER — *The Milleres Tale*, v. 3612.)

Fienus* mentions an instance of a malefactor who was carried out, as he conceived, to execution; and in order thereto his cap was pulled over his eyes, and a cold wet cloth being stuck hastily about his neck, he fell down dead, under the conceit of his decapitation. Charron† records a similar case: A man having his eyes covered to be put to death, as he imagined — being condemned, — and uncovering them again to receive his pardon, was found really dead on the scaffold. It is commonly told, but I am unacquainted with the authority, that a person was directed to be bled to death; his eyes were blinded and he was made to believe, by water trickling down his arm, that the sentence was being carried into effect. The mimicry is said

---

* De Viribus Imaginationibus tractatus. Lugd. Bat. Elzev. 1635, 2 tom. 12mo.

† De la Sagesse, liv. iii., cap. 6.

to have produced his death as effectually as would the real operation. The powers of life were destroyed by the power of his imagination.

Excessive joy has been known to occasion death equally with, nay, more frequently than, fear and terror. Sir Alexander Crichton relates, that "in the year 1544 the Jewish pirate, Sinamus Taffurus, was lying in a port of the Red Sea, called Arsenoe, and was preparing for war, being then engaged in one with the Portuguese. While he was there he received the unexpected intelligence that his son, who in the siege of Tunis had been made prisoner by Barbarossa and by him doomed to slavery, was suddenly ransomed, and coming to his aid with seven ships well armed. The joyful news was too much for him: he was immediately struck as with an apoplexy, and expired on the spot. Valerius Maximus* relates the case of two women, matrons, who died with joy on seeing their sons return safe from battle at the lake Thrases. One died while embracing her son; the other was suddenly surprised by the sight of her son while she was deeply lamenting his supposed death. Sophocles, at an advanced age and in the full possession of his intellectual power, composed a tragedy, which was crowned with such success that he died through joy. Chilon of Lacedemon died from joy whilst embracing his son, who had borne away the prize at the Olympic Games. Juventius Thalma, to

---

* Lib. ix., cap. 12.

whom a triumph was decreed for subjugating Corsica, fell down dead at the foot of the altar at which he was offering up his thanksgiving. Fouquet, upon receiving the intelligence of Louis XIV having restored him to liberty, fell down dead. There are many cases of a similar nature on record.

The cases of sudden death from powerful emotions and unexpected joys or sorrow are numerous in the writings of the ancients. They are doubtless to be attributed to the effects produced by means of the nervous system acting chiefly upon other organs, particularly those which appertain to the sanguiferous system, where either disease or a strong predisposition to it had previously existed. Most of the cases of sudden death which now occur — and they have been lamentably numerous of late — are shown by dissection to arise from disorder of the heart or its large vessels.* Some years

---

* Sympathy appears to exert itself more particularly between the mind and certain organs of the body than with others. Any excitement of the mind quickens the circulation, and occasions the heart to palpitate, that is, to beat quickly and tremulously. Senac (Traité du Cœur, tom. ii., p. 454), quotes a case from Blancard of a person, who, being witness to a dreadful shipwreck, was so operated upon by distress and terror, that palpitation of the heart, succeeded by oppressed breathing, syncope, and death ensued. Upon examination, the heart was found enlarged. The same author mentions other fatal cases occasioned by mental emotions and passions in those in whom, upon examination, the heart was found unnatural and unhealthy. Next to the heart, the organs of digestion seem most susceptible of the effects from mental emotions; and an ingenious writer, Mr. Fletcher, of Gloucester, has ventured to designate the effect of the passions upon the

since it was customary to refer any case of sudden death to apoplexy, and at an earlier period to the effects of fear, joy, or other violent passions. St. Bernard* describes anger, joy, fear, and grief as the wheels of a coach, by which we are carried in this world: "Hæ quatuor passiones sunt tanquam rotæ in curru quibus vehemur in hoc mundo."

Sir Astley Cooper, in his lectures on surgery, was accustomed to relate some instances bearing upon the subject under consideration. The effects of fear in destroying your best efforts to relieve injuries are well known to any surgeon of experience. Sir Astley says that he has often known patients declare, after an accident, that they were sure they should not recover, and they seemed to be deprived of all restorative

---

stomach as a "Mental Indigestion," in contradistinction to that dyspepsia which arises from physical causes. The reciprocity of action between certain passions and certain organs is a subject highly deserving of investigation. Fear, as already stated, produces its most decided effects upon the heart, and it is the especial condition of all who have disease of this organ to be under continual apprehension and dread. Irritability of temper is always consequent upon disordered conditions of the liver and digestive organs. Voltaire knew this well when he said, "Quand vous avez le matin une grâce à demander à un ministre ou à un premier commis de ministre, informez vous adroitement s'il a le ventre libre; il faut toujours prendre *mollia fandi tempora*. Personne n'ignore que notre caractère et notre tour d'esprit dépendent absolument de la garde-robe. Il y a une grande analogie entre les intestines et nos passions, notre manière de penser, notre conduite." Dryden and other eminent authors have not been insensible to the necessity of healthy alimentary function to the free exercise of mental power.

* Serm. 35.

power. I have often witnessed instances of this kind. A gentleman consulted Sir A. Cooper, and he was found to have a stone in his bladder. "I hope not," says he, "for I never can submit to an operation." He returned to the country, and died in a few days after. Mr. Cline operated for a tumour in the breast of a lady. She felt certain the operation would kill her; but she yielded to the solicitations of her friends, submitted to it, and it was performed with great skill, and unattended by anything remarkable. She however died only one hour after the operation; and it was found that she had arranged her family and domestic concerns in such a manner, that no confusion should arise from what she thought her inevitable doom.

A school-mistress, for some trifling offence, most foolishly put a child into a dark cellar for an hour. The child was greatly terrified and cried bitterly. Upon returning to her parents in the evening, she burst into tears, and begged that she might not be put into the cellar; the parents thought this extremely odd, and assured her that there was no danger of their being guilty of so great an act of cruelty; but it was difficult to pacify her, and when put to bed she passed a restless night. On the following day she had fever, during which she frequently exclaimed, "Do not put me in the cellar." The fourth day after, she was taken to Sir A. Cooper, in a high state of fever, with delirium, frequently muttering, "Pray don't put me in the cellar." When Sir Astley inquired the reason, he found that the parents had learnt the punishment to which she had been subjected. He ordered what was likely to relieve her, but she died in a week after this unfeeling conduct.

Another case from the same authority may here be cited. It is the case of a child, ten years of age, who wanted to write her exercise, and, to scrape her slate pencil, went into the school in the dark to fetch her knife, when one of her school-fellows burst from behind the door to frighten her. She was much terrified, and her head ached. On the following day she became deaf, and on the next, so much so as not to hear the loudest talking. Sir Astley saw her three months after this had happened, and she continued in a deplorable state of deafness.

Platerus* relates a case of fatal convulsions produced by terror. Some young girls went one day a little way out of town to see a person who had been executed, and who was hung in chains. One of them threw several stones at the gibbet, and, at last, struck the body with such violence as to make it move; at which the girl was so much terrified, that she imagined the dead person was alive, came down from the gibbet, and ran after her. She hastened home, and not being able to conquer the idea, fell into strong convulsions and died.

An extraordinary case of the effects of fear is recorded by Dr. Bateman.† A middle-aged woman, in previous good health, was thrown into a state of great fright and alarm upon dis-

---

* Observ. lib. i., p. 36.
† Edinb. Med. and Surg. Journal, vol. v., p. 127.

covering in the evening that she had lost her little store of money, the savings of several years, and the next morning she was anasarcous from head to foot. By judicious treatment she recovered.

Convulsions, epilepsy, madness, and idiocy have all been produced by fear and terror. The wife of Schenckius[*] was attacked with epilepsy, from a fright occasioned by a fire. She had previously been in robust health, but at this time was in the last month of pregnancy. She died in twelve hours.

A boy, fifteen years of age, was admitted an inmate of the Dundee Lunatic Asylum, having become imbecile from fright. When twelve years of age he was apprenticed to a light business, and some trifling article being one day missing, he was, along with others, locked up in a dark cellar. The children were much alarmed, and all were let out, with the exception of this poor boy, who was detained until past midnight. He became from this time nervous and melancholy, and sunk into a state of insensibility, from which he will never recover. The missing article was found on the following morning, exculpating the boy from the guilt with which he had been charged. Dr. Scott[†] relates a case of convulsions occasioned by fear, from a butcher-boy running after another, ten years of age, threatening to kill him; and also the case of a girl, eight years of age, in whom,

---

[*] Observ. Medic., lib. i., p. 128.
[†] Edinb. Med. and Surg. Journal, vol. xliii., p. 328.

from panic, inflammation of the membranes of the brain, accompanied by defective sight and hearing, was induced, and proved fatal. The same authority gives also an instance of chorea excited by fear, in a girl of thirteen, from seeing two boys quarrelling in the street.

During the prevalence of cholera, many persons, powerfully impressed by fear of taking the disease, caused such disorder of the system, that in several instances death ensued.* Dr. Crowther, of Wakefield, saw a case of tetanus induced by terror, occasioned by a spectral illusion. Tulpius† relates a case of Volvulus ex Ira, a case of fatal ileus, occasioned by a fit of anger.

Van Swieten‡ mentions the case of a boy attacked with epilepsy, from a dog leaping on him; and the sight of a large dog, or the barking of one, frequently induced a recurrence of the paroxysm.

Dr. Reid witnessed a case in which an attack of epilepsy almost immediately followed a fit of anger; and he has reported§ the case of a woman approaching to absolute blindness, occasioned by fright at witnessing a paroxysm of epilepsy with which her husband was affected in the night. In one eye the vision was completely destroyed; in the other the capacity of seeing was intermittent, "going and coming,"

* Lond. Med. and Phys. Journal, vol. lxviii., p. 340.
† Observ. Med., lib. ii., n. 41.
‡ Comment. in H. Boerhaavii Aphor.
§ Lond. Med. and Phys. Journal, vol. xiv., p. 15.

as she herself described it, "like the sun when a cloud passes over it." The nervous system was otherwise affected, as a certain degree of deafness was also produced by the same cause.

Dr. Erdman, of Dresden, mentions in his 'Medical Observations' a very singular phenomenon which he witnessed in a boy, of a delicate complexion, light hair, and a sanguine temperament. Whenever this boy fell into a passion one half of his face would become quite pale, while the other was very red and heated, and these two colours were exactly limited by a line running down the middle of the forehead, nose, lips, and chin. When this boy had heated himself by any violent exercise, the whole face became equally red.

Fear has been known to produce hydrophobic symptoms. A remarkable case of this kind was submitted in detail to the Royal Academy of Sciences at Paris, in 1823. M. Buisson had attended a woman in hydrophobia; he bled her: his hands were smeared with the blood, and he wiped them with a cloth which had been applied to remove the saliva from the mouth of the patient. M. Buisson had an ulceration upon one of his fingers at the time, which circumstance no doubt dwelt upon his mind. On the ninth day after his attendance he was suddenly seized with a pain in his throat and eyes, the saliva was continually discharging itself from his mouth, the impression of a current of air, the appearance of a shining substance occasioned him painful sensations, his body seemed to him so light that he felt as though he could leap a prodigious height, and he had a desire to bite — not men, but animals and inanimate bodies. He now began to drink with difficulty, and the sight of water was exceedingly distressing to him. He traced the pain of his throat, which recurred every five minutes, as extending from his finger up the arm to the shoulder and neck. He conceived himself labouring under hydrophobia; and horribly impressed by its fatality, he resolved to terminate his existence by stifling himself in a vapour-bath. He caused the temperature of the bath to be raised to 42°, (107° 36″ Fahr.), when he was equally surprised and delighted to find himself completely well. He left the bathing-room, dined heartily, drank more than usual, and remained perfectly free from all complaint.

The 'Journal de Médecine' gives a case of a medical pupil who assisted at a *post-mortem* examination of a case of hydrophobia, and imagined that he had inoculated himself with the disease. He suffered many of the early symptoms of hydrophobia, abandoned himself to despair, and wandered about the streets considering his doom as inevitably fixed. His friends, however, at length succeeded in relieving his depression and restoring him to health.

A singular case of the depressing effects of terror is recorded by Pechlin.* A lady of quality who, in the year 1681, had several times seen, without alarm, the wonderful comet which

* Lib. iii., Obs. 23.

then appeared, was one night tempted to examine it by means of a telescope; the sight of it, however, in this way, terrified her so much that she was with difficulty carried safely home; and, the impression remaining, she died in a few days afterwards.

One of the most remarkable cases of the effect of terror is quoted from Bonetus* by Sir Alexander Crichton. It was a case of catalepsy — a rare disease, in which the action of the will is annihilated by the disordered condition of the brain and nervous system. " George Grokatzki, a Polish soldier, deserted from his regiment in the harvest of the year 1677. He was discovered a few days afterwards, drinking and making merry in a common ale-house. The moment he was apprehended he was so much terrified, that he gave a loud shriek, and immediately was deprived of the power of speech. When brought to a court-martial, it was impossible to make him articulate a word; nay, he then became as immoveable as a statue, and appeared not to be conscious of anything which was going forward. In the prison to which he was conducted he neither ate nor drank; neither did he make any water, nor go to stool. The officers and the priests at first threatened him, and afterwards endeavoured to soothe and calm him, but all their efforts were in vain. He remained senseless and immoveable. His irons were struck off, and he was taken out of the prison, but he did not move. Twenty days and knights

---

* Medic. Septentrion, lib. i., sect. xvi., cap. 6.

were passed in this way, during which he took no kind of nourishment, nor had any natural evacuation; he then gradually sunk and died."

The most singular instance of the power of the will over the functions of the body, and, taken altogether, perhaps the most remarkable case on record, being supported by the testimony of unquestionable authority, is related by Dr. Cheyne in his 'English Malady.' It is the case of the Hon. Colonel Townshend, who for many years had suffered from an organic disease of the kidney, by which he was greatly emaciated. He was attended by Dr. Cheyne, Dr. Baynard, and Mr. Skrine; and these gentlemen were sent for early one morning to witness a singular phenomenon. He told them he had for some time observed an *odd sensation*, by which, if he composed himself, he could die or expire when he pleased, and by an effort come to life again. The medical attendants were averse, in his weak state, to witness the experiment; but he insisted upon it, and the following is Dr. Cheyne's account: "We all three felt his pulse first: it was distinct, though small and thready, and his heart had its usual beating. He composed himself on his back, and lay in a still posture some time; while I held his right hand, Dr. Baynard laid his hand on his heart, and Mr. Skrine held a clean looking-glass to his mouth. I found his pulse sink gradually, till at last I could not feel any by the most exact and nice touch. Dr. Baynard could not feel the least emotion in his heart, nor Mr. Skrine the least soil of breath on the bright mirror he held to his mouth; then each of us by turns examined his arm, heart, and breath; but could not, by the nicest scrutiny, discover the least symptom of life in him. We reasoned a long time about this odd appearance as well as we could, and all of us judging it inexplicable and unaccountable, and finding he still continued in that condition, we began to conclude that he had indeed carried the experiment too far, and at last were satisfied he was actually dead, and were just ready to leave him. This continued about half an hour, by nine o'clock in the morning in autumn. As we were going away we observed some motion about the body, and upon examination found his pulse and the motion of the heart gradually returning; he began to breathe gently and speak softly; we were astonished to the last degree at this unexpected change, and after some further conversation with him, and among ourselves, went away fully satisfied as to all the particulars of this fact, but confounded and puzzled, and not able to form any rational scheme that might account for it. He afterwards called for his attorney, added a codicil to his will, settled legacies on his servants, received the sacrament, and calmly and composedly expired about five or six o'clock that evening."* His body was examined, and all the viscera, with the exception of the right kidney, which was greatly diseased, were found perfectly healthy and natural. This power of the will, to die or live at pleasure, is, perhaps, one of the

* Pages 308-310.

most remarkable phenomena connected with the natural history of the human body. Burton alludes to cases of the same kind, and reports that the celebrated Cardan bragged he could separate himself from his senses when he pleased. Celsus makes reference to a priest who possessed the same extraordinary power.

Hysteria and epilepsy have been repeatedly induced in persons of a nervous temperament from a principle of imitation. The Romans called the latter morbus comitialis, from its having been frequently excited in the Comitia, whence it was afterwards forbidden for any one liable to the disease to enter. Dr. Hardy, of Bath, has recorded some cases of imitative epilepsy.* A healthy young man had the care of an epileptic patient, and he also became epileptic in the highest degree from witnessing the paroxysms. A friend of this young man also became epileptic from occasionally visiting him and observing the fits. Highly excited states of the nervous system, particularly under impressions of a religious nature, have produced convulsions and epileptic attacks; and these occurring amidst assemblies subject to the same influence have occasioned the diseased actions to partake of an epidemic character. A most remarkable instance of this kind occurred in 1814, in Cornwall, and extended its effects over a considerable part of the county and to several thousands of individuals. Mr. Cornish, of Falmouth, gave†

---

* Lond. Med. Gazette, vol. xi., p. 247.
† Lond. Med. and Phys. Journal, vol. xxxi., p. 373.

a curious account of several instances in which he observed the effects of this mental excitement. It took its rise in a Wesleyan chapel in Redruth, and extended to others of the same denomination in Camborne, Helston, Truro, Penryn, and Falmouth. During the time of divine service, a man called out loudly and unexpectedly, "What shall I do to be saved?" and expressed a most alarming apprehension as to the state of his soul. The example thus set was speedily followed, and the individual affected seemed to suffer great bodily pain. This circumstance becoming known, hundreds flocked to the chapel from curiosity, and many became similarly affected. The chapel was kept open for several nights and days, and the manifestations not being checked, but, on the contrary, rather promoted by the preachers, who availed themselves of such an opportunity to convert sinners, the emotion extended itself rapidly. The attacks experienced are described by Mr. Cornish as of a nature, in the first instance, resembling attacks of chorea, which afterwards would assume either the character of hysterical or epileptical attacks, and continue, in some instances, for not less than seventy or eighty hours. Children from six years of age to old men of eighty were thus affected, but the cases were mostly of girls and young women. They were chiefly persons of the lowest class and in deplorable ignorance. Mr. Cornish estimates the number of persons affected as not being fewer than four thousand. He was not acquainted with a single case in which it proved fatal. Similar instances of convulsions, produced by sympathy, are to be found in the 'Statistical account of Scotland," occurring in Angusshire and Lanarkshire: some have also been reported by Dr. Haygarth in North Wales, and by Dr. Roberts in Tennessee.*

* In Pike's 'Voyage up the Mississippi' there is a curious account of the superstitions of the American Indians; and among other things he notices the effects produced by their peculiar dances, to one of which he was an eyewitness. The men and women danced indiscriminately. They were all dressed in their gayest manner; each of them holding a small skin of some kind in their hands. They frequently ran up to, pointed their skin, and puffed with their breath, or blew at each other. The person thus blown on, whether man or woman, would instantly fall, and appear almost lifeless, or in great agony, — would recover slowly, rise, and again join in the dance. This is called their great medicine, or the dance of religion. The bystanders actually believe that something is puffed or blown into each other's body, which produces the falling and other effects which take place. All the Indians are not of the initiated. They must first make presents of forty or fifty dollars value to the society, and give a feast, when they are admitted with great ceremony. Mr. Fraser said he was once in a lodge with some young men, when one of these dancers entered: they immediately threw their blankets over him, and forced him out. On his laughing at them, the young Indians called him a fool, and said he did not know what the dancer could blow into his body.

A gentleman at Abingdon, in Virginia, has also given an account of one of the camp-meetings in the Western States, in which convulsions are frequently excited. He tells us that persons who have been greatly affected at these meetings have been exercised in various ways. They laugh, they sing, they dance; and, as it would appear, all this is involuntarily done, being what the preachers call "religious exercises;" but it is doubtful whether they are not the offspring of free will. There is one species of these "religious exercises" which appears to be involuntary, and that has spread from the camp and other religious meetings in an alarming man-

Dr. Haygarth rendered no little service to his profession, and to mankind, by his able exposition of the quackery of the metallic tractors. At the commencement of the present century a quackery prevailed, in which it was contended that certain diseases could be cured by merely drawing over the parts affected certain pieces of metal called tractors. They were introduced by a person of the name of Perkins. The extraordinary effects reported of their operation were, by some, attempted to be accounted for by a supposed galvanic, electric, or magnetic influence, exerted over the disease by the peculiar composition of the metals of which the tractors consisted; but it is not always found practicable, either in physic or philosophy, to dis-

ner. These are called the "jerks." Some of those affected with this disorder will rise up, and, with their eyes fixed and starting, make their feet roll upor the floor. But generally the person who has this disorder, is vexed with a perpetual convulsive jerking in all his limbs. Some of them are said to have vaulted and appeared as if they would have dashed themselves to pieces, if not prevented. In one man affected with this disorder there were not five seconds of time during which some of his limbs, his back, or his spine, were not drawn with a sudden jerk, in one direction or another. There was a muster of some militia companies, and three or four of the jerkers were in the town, and no sooner did the drums begin to beat than they found themselves so violently jerked, that they were forced to decamp with all practical speed. Several persons have taken this disorder who have no religion at all. Sucking children are reported not to be exempt from it; and a wild young man, either from seeing the jerkers or shaking hands with them, is reported to have taken the disorder with great violence. The jerks were considered as a nervous disease, generally produced by horror very strongly excited.

cover the cause and effect of certain conditions. Dr. Haygarth resolved upon putting the metallic tractors to the test of experiment, and, communicating his intentions to his friend Dr. Falconer, he selected five patients from the General Hospital at Bath, and submitted them to the operation of a pair of false tractors, or such as he had himself made, being composed not of metal but of wood, yet so painted as to resemble the metallic ones in colour. The diseases under which the patients thus selected laboured were various, and of a chronic character, gout and rheumatism; and they had been ill several months. Upon the affected parts being stroked in the lightest manner by these pieces of wood, the patients all declared themselves relieved; three of them were particularly benefited, and one immediately improved so much in his walking that he had great pleasure in exhibiting proofs of the benefit he had received. One said he felt a tingling sensation for two hours. Similar experiments with wood, slate pencil, tobacco pipes, &c., were made at the Bristol Infirmary with the same results;* and the fame attending these cures was so spread abroad, that more patients crowded for relief than time could be afforded to bestow upon them. Men that

---

* Dr. Alderson, physician to the Hull Infirmary, also repeated Dr. Haygarth's experiments, and with the same results. A detail of several cases is given in the London Medical and Physical Journal, (vol. iv., p. 100,) and clearly proves that it remained with the operator either to produce ease or to inflict suffering, according to the manner he pleased to exercise with his patient, through the means of the imagination.

were unable to lift up, or to use their arms in any way, were, after the application of the supposed metallic tractors, speedily enabled to carry coals, and other matters of considerable weight, with comparative ease. The results attending these cases were so remarkable, that nothing short of their having been publicly done and attested by witnesses of unimpeachable veracity could satisfy one of their truth.

The cases recorded by Dr. Haygarth* go far to explain how miraculous cures are to be ascribed to empirical remedies; many of which are composed of substances most inert in their nature. It is the confidence of the quack and the hope of the patient which work the cure. Disease is well known to depress the powers of the understanding as well as the vigour of the muscular system, and will also deprave the judgment as well as the digestion. A sick person is, in particular, extremely credulous about the object of his hopes and fears. Whoever promises him health may easily obtain his confidence, and he soon becomes the dupe of quacks and ignorant pretenders. "Ne vaudroit-il pas mieux qu'il fût dans celles d'un médecin éclairé?"†

Medical faith is a matter of very great importance in the cure of diseases, and Dr. Haygarth was quite justified in expressing his wish never to have a patient who did not possess a suffi-

---

* On the Imagination, as a Cause and as a Cure of Disorders of the Body. Bath, 1800, 8vo.

† Cabanis.

cient portion of it. A doctor being asked the question, why he could not cure his mother-in-law as well as his father? wittily replied, that his mother-in-law had not the same confidence, or rather fancy for him, as his father had, otherwise the cure would have been effected. The administration of new medicines, without possessing anything particularly novel or powerful, will frequently induce an amendment in the disease: this may probably arise, in some instances, from the presence of a new stimulus to which the frame has heretofore not been accustomed; but in the majority of cases it will be found to be the result of an effect of the imagination. Hippocrates admitted that that physician performed most cures in whom the patients placed the greatest reliance. Medicines when prescribed by a physician of celebrity have been known to succeed better in his hands than that of other persons. Where faith is wanting little success is to be expected. The influence of hope is necessary to procure relief, and the alleviation or removal of diseases is in a great number of cases dependent upon the condition of the mind. An agreement between the mind and the body is constant; and Sterne truly though singularly expressed this opinion, when he said, "The body and mind are like a jerkin and a jerkin's lining, rumple the one and you rumple the other."

Dr. Paris* has related an anecdote, communicated to him by the late Mr. Coleridge, which

* Pharmacologia, p. 28.

strikingly illustrates the power of the imagination in relieving disease. "As soon as the powers of nitrous oxide were discovered, Dr. Beddoes at once concluded that it must necessarily be a specific for paralysis; a patient was selected for the trial, and the management of it was intrusted to Sir Humphry Davy. Previous to the administration of the gas, he inserted a small pocket thermometer under the tongue of the patient, as he was accustomed to do upon such occasions, to ascertain the degree of animal temperature, with a view to future comparison. The paralytic man, wholly ignorant of the nature of the process to which he was to submit, but deeply impressed, from the representation of Dr. Beddoes, with the certainty of its success, no sooner felt the thermometer under his tongue than he concluded the *talisman* was in full operation, and in a burst of enthusiasm declared that he already experienced the effect of its benign influence throughout his whole body: the opportunity was too tempting to be lost; Davy cast an intelligent glance at Coleridge, and desired his patient to renew his visit on the following day, when the same ceremony was performed, and repeated every succeeding day for a fortnight, the patient gradually improving during that period, when he was dismissed as cured, no other application having been used."

Professor Woodhouse, in a letter to Dr. Mitchell of New York, has given a recital which also tends to show what singular effects can be caused if the imagination be previously and duly prepared for the production of wonders.

At the time that nitrous oxide excited almost universal attention, several persons were exceedingly anxious to breathe the gas; and the professor administered to them ten gallons of atmospherical air, in doses of from four to six quarts. Impressed with the idea that they were inhaling the nitrous oxide, quickness of the pulse, dizziness, vertigo, tinnitus aurium, difficulty of breathing, anxiety about the breast, a sensation similar to that of swinging, faintness, weakness of the knees, and nausea which lasted from six to eight hours were produced — symptoms entirely caused by the breathing of common air, under the influence of an excited imagination.

The consideration of such cases as those now referred to should lead all who practise medicine to look particularly to the mental condition of their patients. There is no subject of greater importance to the medical man, as well as to the philosopher in general, than the consideration of the influence exerted by the mind upon the vital functions of the body. The operation of the moral feelings and emotions in the production of corporeal disease is far from being yet understood. I have but briefly touched upon it in these pages as a means of explaining many circumstances which have been formerly attributed to miraculous and supernatural causes; and I have given evidence only of those stronger and more remarkable cases or events which have appeared to me to show most conspicuously the connexion I have endeavoured to point out. The minuter shades of disease, produced by mental condition, would, however, form a topic of vast interest and importance to the medical philosopher, and it is very much to be regretted that so little attention has hitherto been paid to the subject. Research, in such a field of inquiry, I doubt not, would display many phenomena, which in ancient times were attributed to celestial or supernatural influence, and latterly, to magnetic and other causes, which might be satisfactorily referred to the operations of the nervous system alone without the supervention of other agency. The *modus operandi* is not understood, and the opinions entertained by physiologists are various. Bichat contended that grief, anger, dread, and melancholy, all acted not upon the brain, but upon the heart and the organs of the circulation, and that whatever lesion in the brain or nervous system could be discovered was dependent upon the intermediate influence of the heart. The influence of the passions in modifying the nutritive processes is indeed very remarkable, and has been characterized in ordinary language. Thus we constantly hear of "pining with envy," being "gnawed by remorse," or "wasted by melancholy." Hence it will be seen how essential it is that medical practitioners should attend with patience to the recital of the maladies of those by whom they are consulted, and cheer their depressed spirits by sympathy and consolation. This can be done without any sacrifice of character or abatement of self-respect and independence.

The instances I have cited are sufficient to show the power of the mind over the body, and the influence it exercises in health and in disease. To apply them to the cases in which charms, &c., have been employed, we must look at the character of the diseases, and we shall not fail to find that all, or nearly all, are such as to be especially under the influence of the nervous and sanguiferous systems. I have no intention of explaining all the narratives I have given in this manner; that would be impossible, and the attempt ridiculous; for I hold with Southey, that "there is no truth, however pure, and however sacred, upon which falsehood cannot fasten, and engraft itself thereon."

The charms for agues, and the number of cures vouched for, we have already seen are most numerous. They are, perhaps, to be attributed to the operation of fear or horror occasioned by their odious and disgustful nature, being composed of spiders, toads, and lizards; or to the confidence reposed in the pomp and ceremony of a magical process, by which tone is imparted to the system. Fear and hope, as Milton has observed, are always concomitant passions.

With regard to pestilential diseases, physicians know that contagion is more likely to prevail among those in whom fear predominates than in others. The hope entertained, by the possession of a charm, to avert pestilence, may have operated in many instances so as to counteract the taking of the plague, for which disease such numerous amulets have been found.

Hemorrhage is known to be suppressed by

fright, which throws back the blood from the extreme branches to the larger vessels about the heart. Syncope produces the same effect.

Epilepsy and other nervous disorders have frequently been produced by fright, and are especially under the control of mental emotions. The sight of a person in an epileptic fit, as already mentioned, has frequently produced the same disease in others who had not before experienced it; and so strong is the principle of imitation in our nature, and so powerfully does it act upon us when weakened by disease, that epilepsy is a disorder not admitted into many of our hospitals. Hysteria may be considered in the same point of view. The relief afforded in these cases, and in others of a convulsive nature by relics of saints, charms, &c., can only be attributed to the prepossession entertained of their efficacy in curing the disease.

Hiccup is a convulsive action, and commonly checked by affecting surprise or alarm.

The cures attributed to the prayers of Prince Hohenlohe were all of cases of a nervous character: palsy, lameness, defect of sight, hearing, &c. Dr. Pfeuffer, the directing physician of the Universal Hospital of Bamberg, in his Psychological and Medical Researches respecting these cases,* asserts that they were all chronic disorders — not one of an acute character. The cures were undertaken without ostentation or mystery, nor was there any particular manipulation exercised. The zeal and energy, and self-confidence

* See Horn's Archives for 1822.

of the prince increased with the various cases that pressed upon him, and the crowd of applicants participated with him in the feeling and excitement. In short, all miraculous cures are of the same description, the disorders are similar, and the effects described are precisely the same. It is faith which works the miracle, and in the Hohenlohe cases depended entirely upon the degree of religious feeling or enthusiasm entertained by the sick.

In the Journal of George Fox* a case of lameness suddenly relieved by an unexpected address under a state of religious ecstasy, is thus recorded: "After some time I went to a meeting at Arn-side, where Richard Myer was. Now he had been long lame of one of his arms; and I was moved of the Lord to say unto him amongst all the people, Prophet Myer, stand up upon thy legs, (for he was sitting down,) and he stood up, and stretched out his arm, that had been lame a long time, and said, 'Be it known unto you, all people, that this day I am healed.' But his parents could hardly believe it; but after the meeting was done, had him aside, and took off his doublet: and then they saw it was true. He came soon after to Swarth-more meeting, and there declared how that the Lord had healed him. Yet after this the Lord commanded him to go to York with a message from him; and he disobeyed the Lord; and the Lord struck him again, so that he died about three-quarters of a year after."

* Vol. i., p. 103, edit. Lond. 1794.

An attentive consideration of the various sympathies would, I doubt not, enable us to explain many of the phenomena that have been recorded, and which, without a due knowledge of the human economy, may justly be looked upon as of a miraculous nature.

ROYAL GIFT OF HEALING.

Malcolm. Comes the king forth, I pray you?
Doctor. Ay, sir: there are a crew of wretched souls,
That stay his cure: their malady convinces
The great assay of art; but at his touch,
Such sanctity hath heaven given his hand,
They presently amend.
Malcolm. I thank you, doctor. [Exit *Doctor.*
Macduff. What's the disease he means?
Malcolm. 'Tis call'd the evil:
A most miraculous work in this good king,
Which often, since my here remain in England,
I have seen him do. How he solicits heaven,
Himself best knows; but strangely-visited people,
All swoln and ulcerous, pitiful to the eye,
The mere despair of surgery, he cures;
Hanging a golden stamp about their necks,
Put on with holy prayers: and 'tis spoken,
To the succeeding royalty he leaves
The healing benediction.
MACBETH, Act iv., Sc. 3.

THE credulity of mankind has never been more strongly displayed than in the general belief afforded to the authenticity of remarkable cures of diseases said to have been effected by the imposition of royal hands. The practice seems to have originated in an opinion that there is something sacred or divine attaching either to the sovereign or his functions. The testimonies offered by writers on this subject, and the number of witnesses recorded, are too great and too indisputable to need reference. No one appears to have questioned the validity of the means, and no one has attempted to explain the results obtained, but in connexion with the sanctity of the operator.

The practice appears to be one of English growth, commencing with Edward the Confessor, and descending only to foreign potentates who could show an alliance with the royal family of England. The kings of France, however, claimed the right to dispense the Gift of Healing, and it was certainly exercised by Philip the First; but the French historians say that he was deprived of the power on account of the irregularity of his life. Laurentius,* first physician to Henry IV, of France, who is indignant at the attempt made to derive its origin from Edward the Confessor, asserts the power to have commenced with Clovis I,† A.D. 481, and says that Louis I, A.D. 814, added to

---

* Laurentius (Andreas) De Mirabili Strumas sanandi vi Solis Galliæ Regibus Christianissimis divinitus concessa. Paris, 1609, 12mo.

† See also Mezeray and Daniel, Histoire de France. Among other stories related of the Holy Oil, the Standard of France, &c., one (according to a MS., No. 2903, art. 45, in the Sloane Collection in the British Museum) is that God gave Clovis (A.D. 496) the gift of curing the king's evil, and that he proved it on Lancier, or Lanciet, his favourite. Another states that "Peter appeared to the monk Brightwold, giving him a cruse of oile, and told him that whome he anointed therewith should be king, and have power to cure the people by his touch, which was done in the person of Edward the Confessor."

the ceremonial of touching, the sign of the cross. Mezeray also says, that St. Louis, through humility, first added the sign of the cross in touching for the king's evil: "D. Ludovicus huic ritui de suo pie addidit signaculum crucis et sequens curatio inquit." Laurentius contends that the power belonged to the kings of France *only ;* and that it descended to them by hereditary right and by sacred unction: "Solis Franciæ Regibus per traducem hæreditariam Regni, et sacram unctionem facultas hæc conceditur." (p. 21.) He reports of Francis I, that when a prisoner in Spain he cured a great number of people of struma. Of this sovereign, Lascaris has written :

"Ergo manu admota sanat Rex Chæradas :* estque
Captivus superis gratus ut ante fuit.
Indicio tali, regum sanctissime, qui te
Arcent, invisos suspicor esse Deis."

This is quoted by Jeremy Collier as an epigram thus :

"Hispanos inter sanat Rex Chæradas, estque:
Captivus, superis gratus ut ante fuit ;"†

which clearly means that a sanative virtue was annexed to his person, and did not disappear with the loss of his liberty. An ingenious and learned friend has thus paraphrased the verses:

* That is, struma, scrofula or king's evil, from χοιρας.
† [Among the Spaniards king Chæradas cures,
  Though a captive, he is still favoured by the Gods.]

> "The king applies his hand, diseases fly,
> And though a captive, still the powers on high
> Regard his touch. This striking proof is giv'n,
> That they who bound him are the foes of Heav'n."

In the church of St. Maclou, in St. Denys, Heylin (Cosmograph., p. 184), says the kings of France, with a fast of nine days and other penances, used to receive the gift of healing the king's evil with nothing but a touch. Philip de Comines states, that the king always confessed before the cure of the king's evil. Butler (Lives of the Saints, vol. viii., p. 394) says, "The French kings usually only perform this ceremony on the day they have received the holy communion." The historians who write under the first two families of the French kings are altogether silent as to the kings' curing the evil by the touching. (Veyrard Trav., p. 109.) Philip of Valois is reported to have cured 1400 people afflicted with the king's evil. Of Louis XIII, it was said that he had assigned all his power to Cardinal Richelieu, except that of curing the king's evil. Carte* says, some of the French writers ascribe the gift of healing to their king's devotion towards the relics of St. Marculf, in the church of Corbigny, in Champagne; to which the kings of France, immediately after their coronation at Rheims, used to go in solemn procession. A veneration was also paid to this saint in England, and a room in memory of him, in the palace of Westminster, has frequently been mentioned in the Rolls

---

* History of England, vol. i., b. iv., sect. 42.

OF HEALING.

of Parliament, and which was called the Chamber of St. Marculf, being, as Carte conjectures, probably the place where the kings used to touch for the evil. This room was afterwards called the Painted Chamber. The French kings practised the touch extensively. Gemelli, the traveller, states, that Louis XIV touched 1600 persons on Easter Sunday, 1686. The words he used were, "Le Roy te touche, Dieu te guerisse.* Every Frenchman received fifteen sous, and every foreigner thirty.† The French kings kept up the practice to 1776.

If credit is to be given to a statement (presently to be noticed) by William of Malmesbury, with respect to Edward the Confessor, we must admit that in England, for a period of nearly 700 years, the practice of the royal touch was exercised in a greater or lesser degree, as it extended to the reign of Queen Anne. It must not, however, be supposed that historical documents are extant to prove a regular continuance of the practice during this time. No accounts whatever of the first four Norman kings attempting to cure the complaint are to be found. In the reign of William III, it was not on any occasion exercised. He manifested more sense than his predecessors, for he withheld from employing the royal touch for the cure of scrofula; and Rapin says, that he was so persuaded he should do no injury to persons afflicted with this distemper by not touching

---

* [The king touches thee, may God cure thee.]
† See Barrington's Observations on the Statutes, p. 107.

them, that he refrained from it all his reign. Queen Elizabeth was also averse to the practice, yet she extensively performed it. It flourished most in the time of Charles II, particularly after his restoration, and a public register of cases was kept at Whitehall, the principal scene of its operation.

EDWARD THE CONFESSOR. The power of Edward the Confessor has been readily admitted. Jeremy Collier,* speaking of the many virtues and miraculous powers of Edward, says, "that this prince cured the king's evil is beyond dispute: and since the credit of this miracle is unquestionable, I see no reason why we should scruple believing the rest." He then quotes William of Malmesbury as his authority, goes on to explain the nature of the disease, and adds, "King Edward the Confessor was the first that cured this distemper, and from him it has descended as an *hereditary miracle* upon all his *successors*. To dispute the matter of fact, is to go to the excesses of skepticism, to deny our senses, and be incredulous even to ridiculousness."

It is unnecessary now to prove the folly of the statements made in relation to this power; they are self-evident to us at this period. If the efficacy of the touch were dependent upon the *hereditary* right of succession, that condition was soon destroyed, for the succession was repeatedly interrupted, yet the power is reported to have remained. Neither did it appertain solely to

---

* Ecclesiastical History of Great Britain, vol. i., p. 225.

those of the Romish faith, for it was practised by Elizabeth; and Carte and Collier relate a story of a Roman Catholic who lived in the time of this Queen. "This person," says Collier, "who was very firm in his communion, happened to be thrown into prison, probably upon the score of his recusancy. Being thrown into prison, I say, he grew terribly afflicted then with the king's evil; and having apply'd himself to physicians, and gone through a long fatigue of pain and expense, without the least success, at last he was touched by the Queen, and perfectly cured. And, being asked how the matter stood with him? his answer was, he was now satisfy'd by experimental proof that the Pope's excommunication of her Majesty signify'd nothing, since she still continued blessed with so miraculous a quality."*

William of Malmesbury† relates several miracles performed by Holy St. Edward, one of which refers to a woman affected with scrofula, which manifested itself by an extraordinary enlargement of the glands of the neck. Admonished in a dream to have the parts affected washed by the king, she entered the palace, and the king himself fulfilling this labour of love, rubbed the woman's neck with his fingers dipped in water. Joyous health followed his healing hand. According to the same authority, Ed-

---

* This story is taken from Dr. Tooker's work Charisma, seu Donum Sanitatis, &c.

† Willielmi Malmesburiensis de Gestis Regum Anglorum, lib. ii., p. 91, edit. Francof. 1601, folio.

ward had often previously cured this complaint in Normandy. The original reads thus:

"Porro ut jam de miraculis dicam; adolescentula juxta parilitatem natalium virum habens, sed fructu conjugii carens, luxuriantibus circa collum humoribus, turpem valetudinem contraxerat, glandulis protuberantibus horrenda. Jussa somnis lavatrinam regis exquirere, curiam ingreditur, rex ipse per se opus pietatis ad implens, digitis aqua intinctis collum pertractat mulieris, medicam dextram sanitas festiva prosequitur, lætalis crusta dissolvitur, ita ut vermibus cum sanie profluentibus, omnis ille noxius tumor recederet. Sed quia hiatus ulcerum fœdus et patulus erat, præcepit eam usque ad integram sanitatem, curialibus stipendiis sustentari; veruntamen ante septimanam exactam ita obductis cicatricibus venusta cutis rediit, ut nihil præteriti morbi discerneres; post annum quoque geminam prolem enixa, sanctitatis EDWARDI miraculum auxit. Multotiens eum in Normannia hanc pestem sedasse ferunt, qui interius ejus vitam noverunt. Unde nostro tempore quidam falsam insinuunt operam, qui asseverant istius morbi curationem non ex sanctitate, sed ex regalis prosapiæ hereditate fluxisse."*

---

* [Moreover I shall now speak of miracles. A young married woman, but childless, was afflicted with swellings about her neck, and fell into bad health. Being commanded in her sleep to inquire for the bath-room of the king, she entered the palace, when the pious king, dipping his hands into the water, and stroking her neck, soon restored her to a happy state of health; the tumours that were filled with worms and corrupt blood bursting and disappearing. But as the sores left wide and disgusting cavities, he ordered her to be supported at the crown's expense till perfectly cured. Before the seventh morning a beautiful new skin appeared, so that no vestiges of the disease could be perceived. A year afterwards she had twins, which added greatly to the sanctity of Edward. It is said by those who knew him intimately, that he frequently cured this complaint in Normandy. Hence in our days those assert falsely, when they say that the cure of this disease is not to be attributed to godliness, but to an hereditary royalty.]

I have extracted the original passage from William of Malmesbury, because it is the earliest mention of the gift of healing by the royal touch. The English historians, following this writer, have repeatedly cited it, but it is remarkable that no other author at or near the time of Edward the Confessor has alluded to the supposed power vested in him. Ingulphus,* abbot of the monastery of Croyland, who lived in his reign, is silent respecting it, although he had personal knowledge of him, and fails not to write his many virtues and his great benefactions to the abbey to which he belonged. Marianus Scotus† the monk of Mentz, and Florence the monk of Worcester,‡ two historians who lived nearer the king's time than William of Malmesbury, are equally silent respecting it; and the bull of the Pope Alexander III, by which Edward was canonized about 200 years after his decease, makes no allusion whatever to any of the cures effected by him through the imposition of hands. Ailred, Alured, or, as Tanner spells his name, Ealred, abbot of Rievaulx, (a Cistercian monastery,) who wrote in 1164, and composed an entire book of the life and miracles of Edward, makes, however, an allusion to the case in which he is reported to have exercised

---

* Rerum Anglicarum Scriptorum Veterum a Gale. Oxon. 1684, tom. i., p. 1. But Ingulphus is not esteemed a high authority by antiquaries.

† Chronica cum M. Poloni supputationibus. Basil, 1559, folio.

‡ Flores Historiarum per Matthæum Wetsmonasteriensem collecti. Francof. 1601, folio.

this power.* These facts might lead one to question the accuracy of William of Malmesbury, and to suppose that he has either been imposed on, or for some unknown object of fraud the statement has been given. Peter of Blois† has been mentioned as one of the earliest to repeat the relation; and it is very easy to conceive how readily it would be credited, and how eagerly it would be transmitted after an authority so deservedly great had placed faith in the circumstance. He was archdeacon of Bath and chaplain to Henry II.

There are no particulars given beyond those I have already mentioned, as to the means employed by Edward the Confessor, nor is there any reference made to any piece of money bestowed at the time. But in the Computus Hospitii of Edward I, preserved among the records in the tower, a small sum of money, (gold medal,) as given by the king to the applicants, is there frequently mentioned. Dr. Plot, in his 'Natural History of Oxfordshire," (tab. xvi., fig. 5,) figures a piece of gold found in St. Giles's Fields, in the suburbs of Oxford, having the initial E. C., and furnished with two holes, supposed to be for the purpose of affixing a riband; and he has presumed this to be a touching piece of the Confessor. The piece of gold alluded to was impressed only on one side, and was most

---

* Vita Sancti Edwardi Regis et Confessoris in Historiæ Anglicanæ Scriptores X, a Twysden. Lond. 1652, 2 vols. folio. De Glandibus et Vermibus regio tactu à quadam fœmina expulsis. p. 390.

† Epist. CL. ad Clericos Aulæ Regiæ, p. 335, n. 6.

probably an amulet. The initials cannot have been those of Edward, as in his lifetime he did not enjoy the title of confessor — that was a distinction given to him after his decease.*

Prior to Charles II, no particular coin appears to have been executed to be given at the time of healing. His touching pieces are not uncommon; and specimens of his reign and of that of James II and of Anne are to be found in the British Museum. Pinkerton† classes the English touch-

---

* No regular gold coinage deserving the name of currency in England issued forth before the age of Edward III. There is, however, extant one gold piece of Edward the Confessor which there is no reason to believe false, and which is said to have been found in a church: it may have been a piece for an offering or present, as one only is known. It is supposed not to have been a coin, although struck from the same die as the silver pennies; it is a gold penny, never apparently intended for general circulation. Three gold pennies of Henry III are known, and these have also been conjectured to be pieces for presents, not coins in circulation. M. Adrien de Longpérier lately communicated to the Numismatic Society an account of a very remarkable gold coin of Offa. This coin bears on one side, in Arabic, "In the name of God was coined this Dinar, in the year 157." In the centre, "Mahomed is the Apostle of God," in three lines, between which are the words OFFA REX. The reverse is inscribed "Mahomet is the Apostle of God, who sent him with the doctrine and true faith, to prevail over every religion." In the centre, "There is no other God but the one God; he has no equal." There are faults in the orthography of the inscription, which the writer ascribes to the ignorance of the artist, who probably copied it from a Mussulman Dinar, being unacquainted with the Arabic language. The writer is of opinion that this dinar may have been brought into Europe by trade, or by the Arabs who fled in 169 (A.D. 785) from the religious persecutions of the Khahlif Hadi.

† Essay on Medals. Lond. 1808, 8vo., vol. ii., p. 71.

pieces with silver counters; they commonly bear St. Michael and the Dragon on one side, and a ship on the other, as in the accompanying plate,* engraved from gold specimens in the British Museum. Figures 1 and 2 represent a piece of the time of Charles II; figures 3 and 4 a similar one of James II; and figures 5 and 6 another of Queen Anne. Pinkerton also says there were touch-pieces of the Pretenders. Probably that represented in figures 7 and 8, from a specimen in the British Museum, is of this description.

HENRY II. From the time of Edward the Confessor to that of Henry II, I can find no authority for this practice by the sovereigns of England. This monarch is, however, alluded to by Peter of Blois, his majesty's chaplain, who attests both the touching and the cure.

JOHN, EDWARD I. Gilbertus Anglicus, the author of a 'Compendium Medicinæ,' the first practical writer on medicine in Britain, and the first English physician who had the hardihood to expose the ignorance and absurdities of the monks, who then chiefly engrossed the practice of medicine, is, stated, upon the authority of Bale, to have lived in the reign of King John, and is placed by him in the year 1210. His work, however, contains references to the writings of Averhöes, the Arabian physician, which were not translated before the middle of the thirteenth century; and it is probable, therefore, that he lived in the time of Edward I, for whose

---

* See Frontispiece.

practice in the touching for the evil he becomes the authority. He asserts the practice to be an ancient one, and tells us that the disease is called the king's evil, because kings cure it.

EDWARD II. John of Gaddesden, a writer of the fourteenth century, who flourished in 1320, and was of Merton College, Oxford, the first English physician employed at court, and extolled by Chaucer as the most illustrious among writers on medicine, treats of scrofula;* and after enumerating various methods of treatment, recommends that in the event of their failure to cure the disease, the patient should repair to the king, to be touched: "Si hæc non sufficiant, vadat ad Regem ut eum tangat atque benedicat; quia iste morbus vocatur regius; et ad hunc valet contactus serenissimi regis Anglorum."

EDWARD III, RICHARD II. Bradwardine,

---

* Praxis Medica, Rosa Anglica dicta, tom. ii., p. 981. Edit. Augustæ Vindelicorum, 1595, 4to. This work is chiefly collected from the Arabian writers, yet the author has been highly praised by Conringius and Leland, the latter especially lauding his erudition and pronouncing him to be the most ingenious man of his age. Such, however, was not the opinion of Guido de Cauliaco, who, in allusion, to this work, pointedly says, "Last of all arose the *Scentless* Rose of England, in which, on its being sent to me, I hoped to find the odour of sweetness; but, instead of that, I only encountered the fictions of Hispanus, of Gilbert, and of Theodoric." "Ultimo insurrexit una *Fatua* Rosa Anglicana, quæ mihi missa fuit, et visa credidi in ea invenire odorem suavitatis, sed inveni fabulas Hispani, Gilberti, et Theodorici." The severity of this judgment is irreconcileable with justice. The book is, however, a very singular compound of the dissimilar subjects of poetry, philology, physic, surgery, physiognomy, cosmetics, and cookery.

archbishop of Canterbury, lived in the reigns of Edward III and Richard II, dying in 1348. He gives testimony to the antiquity of the practice, and appealing to its truth, says, "Quicunque negas miracula Christiane, veni et vide ad oculum, adhus istis temporibus in locis sanctorum per vices miracula gloriosa."* †

Henry IV, V, VI. Sir John Fortescue, Lord Chief Justice of the King's Bench in the time of Henry IV, and afterwards Chancellor to Henry VI, in his 'Defence of the Title of the House of Lancaster,' now in the Cotton Library, and written just after Henry the Fourth's accession to the crown, represents the privilege of touching for the evil as a practice from time immemorial belonging to the kings of England; and he attributes the derivation of the power to the unction of their hands employed at their ceremonial of coronation. "Reges Angliæ in ipsa unctione sua talem cœlitus gratiam infusam recipiunt, quod per tactum manuum suarum unctarum infectos morbo quodam, qui vulgo *regius morbus* appellatur, mundant et curant, qui alias dicuntur incurabiles."‡

Henry VII. This monarch was a great observer of religious forms, and was the first sove-

* In Libro de Causâ Dei, lib. i., cap. 1, corol. pars. 32, p. 39.

† [Whoever thou art, O Christian, who denyest these miracles, come and be an eyewitness of their truth, &c.]

‡ [The kings of England at the time of unction receive such a divine power, that, by the touch of their hands, they can cleanse and cure those who are otherwise considered incurable of a certain disease, commonly called the king's evil.]

reign, who established a particular service of ceremony to be employed at the healings. Mr. Beckett* thinks he can trace the ceremony established by Henry VII, to have been derived from a very old MS. exorcism, used for the dispossessing of evil spirits. The service has been altered at different times, though the variations are not great. The variations are to be found in the reigns of Charles II and of Queen Anne. In the Book of Common Prayer, of the latter reign, the service is printed. The form of prayer used at the healing was separately printed originally, and it was reprinted among the additions to L'Estrange's 'Alliance of Divine Offices.' Bishop Kennett also preserved it in his register, p. 731, with this remark, that "he thinks this was the only office changed by King James II, and performed by his own priests," and "that it was restored by Queen Anne with very little correction."

In the reign of Henry VII, the presentation of a piece of gold was first generally introduced. It probably descended from a practice common in the time of Edward III, whose rose-noble had, on one side the king's image in a ship, and on the reverse a religious inscription, "Jesus autem transiens per medium eorum ibat;"' and these coins are said to have been worn as amulets to preserve from danger in battle. Many coins of this description are to be found in the collection

* A Free and Impartial Enquiry into the Antiquity and Efficacy of Touching for the Cure of the King's Evil; by William Beckett. Lond. 1772, 8vo., p. 52, and Appendix, No. VI., p. 14.

of the British Museum and in other cabinets, having sentences from scripture of a holy character, which doubtless were employed with the same intent. The *angel-noble* of Henry VII* appears to have been the coin given, as it was of the purest gold; it was the coin of the time, and not made especially for this purpose. It bore the inscription, "*Per Cruce tua salva nos xpe rede;*" but in the time of Elizabeth this was altered to "*A Domino factum est istud et est mirabile in oculis nostris.*" After the reign of Elizabeth it was found necessary to reduce the size of the coin, so great were the numbers that applied to be touched, and the inscription was therefore reduced to that of *Soli Deo gloria*, which continued to be the case to the time of Queen Anne.

HENRY VIII. Polydore Virgil, who lived in the reigns of Henry VII and VIII, describes the disease and attests the practice in his day. "Solebat rex Edovardus divinitus solo tactu sanare strumosos, hoc est, strumam patientes: est enim struma morbus, quem Itali scrophulam vulgo vocant, à scrophis, quæ ea mala scabie afflictantur, id est humor, in quo subtus concretæ quædam ex pure et sanguine, quasi glandulæ oriuntur, ac plurimum per pectus, et guttur serpit. Quod quidem immortale munus, jure

---

* The angel is represented standing with both feet on the dragon. (See Ruding's Annals of the Coinage of Britain, &c., vol. v., p. 223, Pl. IV., No. 7.) Fabian Phillips (on Purveyance, p. 257) says that the angels issued by the kings of England on occasion of the touchings amounted to a charge of 3000*l.* per annum.

quasi hæreditario, ad posteriores reges manavit: nam reges Angliæ etiam nunc tactu, ac quibusdam hymnis non sine cærimoniis prius recitatis, strumosos sanant."* †

ELIZABETH. I have already alluded to a case of evil,‡ touched by the Queen Elizabeth; but the chief evidence of Her Majesty's exercise of this privilege is afforded by a publication from which Carte and Collier had extracted the case before mentioned, a work by the Rev. Dr. William Tooker, chaplain to the queen and canon of Exeter, (where he was born,) and afterwards dean of Lichfield. He died in 1620, having published his work whilst queen's chaplain, and it is entitled, " Explicatio totius Qæstionis de mirabilium sanitatum gratia, in qua præcipue agitur de Solemni et sacra curatione strumæ, cui Reges Angliæ, rite inaugurati, divinitus medicati sunt," Lond. 1597, 4to. This is an historical defence of the power of our kings in curing what is commonly called the king's evil. He flatters her majesty upon her extraordinary abilities in *touching* or *healing*, for these words were synonymous. He attributes the power to all Christian kings, and is displeased with those who are content to derive it from an authority

---

* Historiæ Anglicæ, lib. xxvi., p. 187. Lugd. Batav. 1649, 8vo.

† [King Edward used to cure the evil merely by the touch. The evil is a disease which the Italians call scrofula, from *scrofa*, a sow, which animal is afflicted with a complaint, that engenders kernels filled with matter and blood, which spread over the breast and throat.]

‡ See page 159.

so recent as Edward the Confessor. In this work, which is now of great rarity, the reverend doctor declares that "the queen never refused touching any body that applied to her for relief, after it had appeared, upon a strict inquiry and examination made by her physicians and surgeons, and by a certificate under their hands, that the complaint of the diseased was really the *king's evil*, and was of so virulent a nature that there were no hopes of its being cured by physicians, or else the sick persons so very indigent, that, not being able to apply to physicians for remedies, they had no resource left but in her royal goodness. This was done to prevent any impositions being made on her sacred touch by any other foul disease; every person admitted to be touched being obliged to pass such examination, and to take with them a ticket from the physician and surgeon by whom they were examined."

Laurentius, as already mentioned, denies to the kings of England the power of healing the evil by the touch, and ascribes it only to those of France. The Rev. Dr. Tooker gives it to the kings and queens of England and denies it to those of France. Laurentius was first physician in ordinary to Henry IV of France, and Tooker was chaplain to Queen Elizabeth. Fuller (Church History, p. 147), quaintly, and in his usual dry style, observes, in allusion to the appointment of Laurentius, that he " had his judgment herein bowed awry with so weighty a relation; flattery being so catching a disease, wherewith the best doctors of physick may sometimes be infected." Tooker he describes as crying quits with him, and admitting the kings of France only to have enjoyed the power *per aliquam Prcpaginem*, by sprig of right, derived from the primitive power of our English kings, under whose jurisdiction most of the French provinces were once subjected. Fearful of enlarging to too great an extent on this subject, Fuller stops short in his discourse, which he says, " begins to bunch and swell out, and some," he adds, " will censure this digression for a *struma*, or tedious exuberance, beyond the just proportion of our history; wherefore, no more hereof: onely I will conclude with two prayers; extending the first to all good people, that Divine Providence would be pleased to preserve them from this painful and loathsome disease. The second I shall confine to myself alone (not knowing how it will suit with the consciences and judgments of others), yet so as not excluding any who are disposed to join with me in my petition; namely, that if it be the will of God to visit me (whose body hath the seeds of all sicknesse and soul of all sins), with aforesaid malady, I may have the favour to be touched of his majesty, the happiness to be healed by him, and the thankfulness to be gratefull to God the author, and God's image, the instrument of my recovery."

William Clowes, surgeon to Queen Elizabeth, denominates scrofula " the *King's* or the *Queen's* Evil: a disease repugnant to nature: which grievous malady is known to be miraculously cured and healed by the sacred hands of the queen's most royall majesty, even by divine inspiration and wonderfull worke and power of God, above man's skill, arte, and expectation. Through whose princely clemency, a mighty number of her majestyes most royal subjects, and also many strangers borne, are dayly cured and healed, which otherwise would most miserably have perished."*

Although a firm believer in the power of the queen over this disease, he yet scouts those who " seriously follow exorcismes and the illusions of certaine charmes of clowtes and rags, which is very inhumane and barbarous: never practised, neither written of, nor allowed by any learned phisition or chirurgeon that ever I yet heard or read of."† From this author's account, it is evident that the queen touched an immense number of persons, though she is reported to have been averse to the practice, and for some time to have even discontinued it. In one of her majesty's progresses in Gloucestershire, she was so tired by the importunity of persons to be touched that she told the people " God only could relieve them from their complaints."

Richard Smith, the titular bishop of Calcedon, says that Elizabeth's cases were cured by giving the sign of the cross, and that from her time to that of James II, this practice was discontinued, but there is no foundation whatever for the opinion expressed by the bishop.

* A Right Frutefull and approoved Treatise, for the Artificiall Cure of that Malady called in Latin, Struma, and in English, the Evill, cured by Kinges and Queenes of England. Lond. 1602, 4to., Pref. Epist.
† Ibid., p. 19.

JAMES I. This sovereign must also have exercised the touch, as a proclamation, bearing date March 25th, 1616, is extant, forbidding patients to approach the royal person during the summer.

In Nichols's 'Progresses,'* we read that "on the 3d Nov., the king knighted, at Whitehall, Sir Edward Stafford; and the Turkish ambassador had his publique audience of his majesty in the banquetting house, purposely hung for him with rich hangings, when his majesty touched one of his followers, said to be his son, for the cure of the king's evil, using at it the accustomed ceremony of signing the place infected with the crosse, but no prayers before or after."† And in the collection at the State Paper Office I have found three letters bearing upon this subject, from which I have made the following extracts:

Extract of a letter from John Chamberlain to Sir Dudley Carleton, ambassador at the Hague. Dated, 7th Nov., 1618:

"On Tuesday the Turkish Chiaus went to the court, but how he carried himself, or what his errand is, I know not: but we say you are likely to have him in Holland."

Extract of a letter from Mr. Pory to the same. Dated London, 7th Nov., 1618:

"On Sunday, the new Venetian ambassador, Signor Donati, had his first audience, and on Tuesday the Turkish Chiaus, who means to

---

* Vol. iii., p. 494, Reign of James I.
† Finetti Philoxenis, p. 58.

have a bout also with Holland. His speech to the king (as my Lord Chancellor told me), was:—Sultan Osman, my great master hath sent your majesty a thousand commendations and a thousand good wishes, both to your majesty and to the prince your sonne, and hath commanded me to present unto you these his Imperial letters. In fine, after his majesty had asked him many questions, the Turke said his sonne was troubled with a disease in his throat, whereof he understood his majesty had the guifte of healing; wherat his majesty laughed heartily, and as the young fellowe came neare him he stroked him, with his hande, first on the one side and then on the other: marry without Pistle or Gospell."

Extract of a letter from the same to the same. Dated London, 14th Nov., 1618.

"The Turkish Chiaus is shortly coming for the Hagh. On Tuesday last he took leave of the king, and thanked his majesty for healing his sonne of the kinges evill; which his majesty performed with all solemnity at Whitehall on Thursday was sevenight."

CHARLES I. This sovereign touched for the evil, and substituted in some cases the giving a piece of silver instead of gold. In Aubrey's 'Collection of Letters' there is one from Dr. Hickes to Dr. Hearne, in which reference is made to a case successfully touched by Charles I, when he was a prisoner in Holmby House. In Whitelock's 'Memorials of English Affairs,' (p. 244, ed. 1732,) under date of April 22, 1647, it is recorded that "Letters informed the great resort of people to the king to be cured of the king's evil, whereupon the House ordered a declaration to be drawn *to inform the people of the superstition of being touched by the king for the evil.* And a letter of thanks ordered to the commissioners at Holmby."

Badger says* that this king "excelled all his predecessors in the divine gift; for it is manifest beyond all contradiction, that he not only *cured* by his sacred *touch*, both with and without gold, but likewise perfectly effected the same cure by his prayer and benediction only."

In the State Paper Office there are preserved no less than eleven proclamations issued in the reign of Charles I, relating to the cure of the king's evil. The first bears the date of June 18, 1626, and is entitled 'A Proclamation for the better ordering of those who repayre to the Court for their Cure of the Disease called the King's Evill.' It ordains that in future the seasons for such purpose should be at Easter and Michaelmas; the latter being substituted for Whitsuntide, as formerly practised, and this "as times more convenient, both for the temperature of the season and in respect of any contagions which may happen in this neere accesse to his majesties person." It also orders that those who repair to the court should bring with them certificates under the hands of the parson, vicar, or minister and churchwardens of those parishes where they dwell, as to not having be-

---

* Cases of Cures of the King's Evil, perfected by the Royal Touch. Lond. 1748, 8vo., p. 27.

fore been touched for the disease. And the proclamation is directed to be affixed in every market town. No. 2, June 17, 1628, is to the same effect, and forbidding any to repair to the court before Michaelmas. No. 3, April 6, 1630, is of the same purpose. No 4, March 25, 1631, is to the same intent, adding that "the danger being now visible to have any concourse of people in this spring or summer time to have resort to this citie of London, the place of his usual accesse, or to his court or royal person." No 5, October 13, 1631, states that "His most excellent majestie (now considering that the danger of the infection of the plague is very much dispersed in divers counties of this kingdome), commands that none presume to repair to the court to be healed before the 15th of December next ensuing; and in case the infection should continue or increase — which God of his mercie divert — his majesty will in the meantime signify and declare his royal will and pleasure by proclamation," &c. No. 6, November, 8, 1631, is entitled 'A Proclamation inhibiting the resort of his majesties people to the court for cure of the king's evill until the middle of Lent, and to restraine the accesse of others from infected places." It alludes to the former proclamation, and adds that, "As it hath not yet pleased Almighty God to withdraw his hand, but that the infection is still much dispersed, they are forbidden to resort to the court until the middle of Lent next; at which time he purposeth (if God shall be so pleased), to admit them to his presence, and for them to doe as hath been used, strictly charging all his officers and ministers whom it shall concerne, that they make stay of as many as they shall find a travailing, or preparing themselves to his majestie for cure of that infirmitie, and to turn them and others whom they shall find to come from places infected to the places of their residence, not suffering them to approach to his majesties presence or his court, or the court or household of his dearest consort the Queene, as they will avoid his majesties displeasure and the paines by his lawes ordained against contemners of his command." No. 7, June 20, 1632: the infection still prevailing, persons were forbidden to apply until Christmas next. No. 8, April 20, 1634, directed that none should "repayre to the court untill the Feast of All Saints next comming." No. 9, December 14, 1634, is a proclamation putting off the time announced, in the following words: "Yet now, having taken into his royal consideration the present general dispersion and overspreading of the small-pox throughout all parts of this kingdom, and the danger that may ensue to his majesties person and household by the accesse and confluence of those people to his court for cure;" it forbids any to appear before Easter next. No 10, July 28, 1635, is a proclamation announcing the times to be as heretofore — Easter and Michaelmas; and directs it to be read twice a year — at Shrovetide and Bartholomewtide, as well as being affixed in every market town. No. 11, September 3, 1637, puts off the healing at Michaelmas next, "the infection still prevailing, upon pain of his majesties high indignation, and such further punishments as shall be meet to be inflicted for the neglect and contempt of his majesties royal commands herein."

In the 'Mercurius Aulicus' for Sunday, March 26, 1643, we read: "His majesty caused an order (which had been signed and printed the day before) to be posted on the court gates and all the posts and passages into the citie of Oxford, prohibiting all such as were troubled with the disease called the king's evil to repair into the court for the cure thereof, at the feast of Easter, now approaching, or at any other time hereafter, till the Michaelmas next."

The Rev. Mr. Peck* relates a case of cure effected by the king, which he found in Oudart's MS. Diary of the Treaty of Newport, in the reign of Charles.

CHARLES II. In no reign did the practice prevail to such an extent as in that of this sovereign, and it is not a little remarkable that more people died of scrofula, according to the Bills of Mortality, during this period than any other. This may probably have arisen from a reliance placed on the royal power, by which other more natural aid was neglected to be sought after.

Parish registers were kept, during this period, of such cases as had received certificates and were touched for the king's evil. Lysons refers to one of these at Camberwell,† and gives extracts from it. He only knew of this one, but

---

* Desiderata Curiosa, vol. ii., lib. x., p. 7.
† Environs of London, vol. i., p. 61.

there was another in the parish of Stanton, St. John, near Oxford, another in the parish of Wadhurst, in Sussex, (1684,) and probably many others yet unnoticed. In the ordinances made by King Charles II for the government of his household, published from the MS., under the royal sign manual, in the library of Thomas Astle, Esq., p. 352, we read: "And whereas many infirme people resort for healing to our court, and first for their probation use to flock to the lodgings of our chirurgions within our house, (which is not only noysome, but may be very dangerous in time of infection); we command that henceforth no such resort be permitted within our house, but that probation of such persons as are to be brought to our presence be made in other places, without admitting any into the house till the day for healing be appointed by us, and order given for the same by our lord chamberlaine or vice chamberlaine, who only are to move us therein."

Pepys has two notices in relation to the touching during this reign. "June 23, 1660: To my lord's lodgings when Tom Grey come to me, and there staid to see the king touch people for the king's evil. But he did not come at all, it rayned so; and the poor people were forced to stand all the morning in the rain in the garden. Afterward he touched them in the banquetting-house."*

"April 13, 1661: I went to the banquet-house, and there saw the king heale, the first time that

---

* Diary, vol. i., p. 59.

ever I saw him do it; which he did with great gravity, and it seemed to me to be an ugly office and a simple one."* There is also a Proclamation preserved in the State Paper Office, of the date of July 4, 1662, ordering that from henceforth the times for healing should be "from the feast of All Saints, commonly called Alhallontide, to a week before Christmas, and in the moneth before Easter."

John Browne, one of the surgeons in ordinary to Charles II, and surgeon to his majesty's hospital, published, in 1684, a curious work, entitled "Adenochoiradelogia: or an Anatomick-Chirurgical Treatise of Glandules and Strumaes, or King's Evil Swellings." He appears to have been the best fitted advocate for the royal gift of healing that could be found, as he enjoyed full belief in the divinity of kings, and his excessive adulation of their power seems to have been most acceptable to Charles II, inasmuch as in the royal permission prefixed to the work, the king expressly says it is a performance "to our great liking and satisfaction." The work is also dedicated to the king, and the author lays his "Anatomical Exercitations prostrate at his Majesty's feet, humbly imploring his sacred touch."

Browne's book is divided into three parts: the first, *Adenochoiradelogia*, treats of the anatomy and offices of the glandular system; the second, *Chœradelogia*, of the nature of strumaes, or king's evil swellings; and the third, *Charisma Basili-*

---

* Ibid., vol. i., p. 100.

con or the royal gift of healing strumaes, or king's evil swellings, by contact, or imposition of the sacred hands of our kings of England and of France, given them at their inaugurations. Struma, or scrofula, is alluded to, in the dedication of the second part to the Earl of Arlington, the lord chamberlain, as a disease with which "the court is extremely visited, and a multitude of poor people are said to give his majesty trouble too oft for curing their diseases they will have to be evil, although not really so, save only in their own conjectures," a circumstance which probably admits of a ready explanation when it is considered that the present of a piece of gold to work the charm accompanied the imposition of hands.

Doubtless, to abridge the royal manual labour, and diminish also the expense attendant upon its operation, the surgeon in ordinary (who speaks of himself as evermore having been conversant in chirurgery, almost from his cradle, being the sixth generation of his own relations all eminent masters of their profession) received "the royal command to attend at all healings, (although the meanest,) and seeing several thousands approach the royal presence for ease and cure, he thought it his duty, as well as his zeal, to search into the roads and circuits of the evil which was seen so frequently to visit the court;" and he adds, "the only reason which invited me to this undertaking was partly intended to prevent the tedious journeys of many poor people who unhappily have undertaken the same upon the pretence of their being troubled with this disease, and partly to secure his Majesty from being cheated of his gold." The third part, treating especially of the royal touch, is inscribed to the Lord Bishop of Durham, clerk of the closet to his Majesty, whose duty it was to present the pieces of gold used at the healings.

The author traces the gift of healing from our Saviour to the Apostles, and thence by a continual line of Christian kings and governors, holy men, commencing with Edward the Confessor, whom he regards as the first curer of struma by contact or imposition of hands. John Browne is a great stickler for the limitation of the power of healing by the royal touch to the kings of England; and although he cannot deny to the French king the possession of this faculty, he contends that it has been derived from the English by "sprig of right." With regard to the manner in which the healing was performed, he tells us, that the surgeon having discovered the disease by examination, he grants a certificate to that effect; and tickets being delivered out to the afflicted, they are then presented to his majesty on the surgeon's knee, and he thus delivers every sick person to the king's sacred hand to be touched. The clerk of his majesty's closet first presents a bit of gold to the king, which he receives from the keeper of the closet, upon whose arm the gold medals ready strung are hanging, whilst the chaplains read the ceremonies and prayers appointed for the purpose, in all which (it is said) "is shown the great charity, piety, clemency, and humility of our dread sovereign; the admirable effects and wonderful events of his royal cure throughout all nations, where not only English, Dutch, Scotch, and Irish have reaped ease and cure, but French, Germans, and all countreyes whatsoever, far and near, have abundantly seen and received the same; and none ever, hitherto, I am certain, mist thereof, unless their little faith and incredulity starved their merits, or they received his gracious hand for curing another disease, which was not really evermore allowed to be cured by him; and as bright evidences hereof, I have presumed to offer that some have immediately upon the very touch been cured; others not so easily quitted from their swellings till the favour of a second repetition thereof. Some also, losing their gold, their diseases have seized them afresh, and no sooner have these obtained a second touch, and new gold, but their diseases have been seen to vanish, as being afraid of his majesties presence; wherein also have been cured many without gold; and this may contradict such who must needs have the king give them gold as well as his touch, supposing one invalid without the gift of both. Others seem also as ready for a second change of gold as a second touch, whereas their first being newly strung upon white riband, may work as well (by their favour). The tying the Almighty to set times and particular days is also another great fault of those who can by no means be brought to believe but at Good Friday and the like particular seasons this healing faculty is of more vigour and efficacy than at any other time, although performed by the same hand. As to the giving of gold, this only shows his majesties royal well-wishes towards the recovery of those who come thus to be healed. This gold being hereat given as a token of his sacred favour, and pledge of his best desires for them."

Prayers were read during the whole of the ceremony, and upon the laying of the king's hands upon them was recited, "They shall lay their hands on the sick and they shall recover." When finished, the lord and the vice-chamberlain, or other two nobles, bring to the king linen and a base and ewer to wash his hands, and he then takes leave of the people. Evelyn records an account of one of these meetings for healing which agrees generally with the preceding statement. It runs thus:

"6 July, 1660. His majestie began first to *touch for ye evil*, according to costome, thus: his ma^tie sitting under his state in ye banquetting house, the chirurgeons cause the sick to be brought or led up to the throne, where they kneeling, ye king strokes their faces or cheeks with both his hands at once, at which instant a chaplaine in his formalities says, 'He put his hands upon them and he healed them.' This is said to every one in particular. When they have ben all touch'd they come up againe in the same order, and the other chaplaine kneeling, and having angel gold strung on white ribbon on his arme, delivers them one by one to his ma^tie, who puts them about the necks of the touched as they passe, whilst the first chaplaine repeats, 'That is ye true light who came into ye world.' Then followes an epistle (as at first

OF HEALING.

a gospell) with the liturgy, prayers for the sick, with some alteration; lastly, ye blessing; and then the lo. chamberlaine and comptroller of the household bring a basin, ewer and towel, for his ma^{tie} to wash."*

The numbers subjected to the royal touch in the reign of Charles II are almost incredible. From a register kept at Whitehall the king appears to have had more patients than all the physicians of his realm. Some were, doubtless, really diseased; but many came for the love of gold, and others from curiosity. The gold was the powerful incentive with many, and instances of attempts to obtain a second piece are narrated. Touching pieces, as they were called, were to be found in the goldsmith's shops, and means were rendered necessary to prevent imposture. The surgeons were required to give certificates to the applicants for relief. According to the Parliamentary Journal for July 2–9, 1660, "The kingdom having been for a long time troubled with the evil, by reason of his majesty's absence, great numbers have lately flocked for cure. His sacred majesty, on Monday last, touched 250 in the banquetting house; among whom, when his majesty was delivering the gold, one shuffled himself in, out of an hope of profit, which had not been stroked, but his majesty quickly discovered him, saying, 'This man hath not yet been touched.' His majesty hath, for the future, appointed every Friday for the cure, at which 200, and no more, are to be

---

* Evelyn's Memoirs, vol. i., p. 323.

presented to him, who are first to repair to Mr. Knight, the king's surgeon, being at the Cross Guns in Russell Street, Covent Garden, over against the Rose Tavern, for their tickets. That none might lose their labour, he thought fit to make it known, that he will be at his home every Wednesday and Thursday, from two to six o'clock, to attend that service; and if any persons of quality shall send to him, he will wait upon them at their lodgings, upon notice given to him."

The giving of the gold was esteemed a token of the king's good will and a pledge of his majesty's best wishes for the recovery of such as came to be healed. It was not regarded as absolutely necessary to the cure, for silver in some few instances was employed with apparently equal benefit. The sovereign power of gold, however, was distinctly admitted, as the disease is reported to have returned in some cases upon the medal being lost, and of being again subdued upon the presentation of a second piece.

Charles II had a respite from practice for two years during the time of the plague, either by his removal from the metropolis or by fear of the epidemic. The register kept by the serjeant and keeper of his majesty's closet belonging to the Chapel Royal, (Thomas Haynes, Esq., and Mr. Thomas Donkley,) gives no enumeration of cases during the years 1665 and 1666, in which time the plague raged grievously. The register extends from May, 1662, to April, 1682, and gives a number of persons touched by the king for the evil, amounting to 92,107.

Fixed days appear, by a proclamation made by the king and council at the court of Whitehall, January 9, 1683, to have been then determined upon, it being ordered that "the times of public healings shall from henceforth be from the feast of All Saints, commonly called Alhallow-tide, till a week before Christmas; and after Christmas until the 1st day of March, and then to cease till the Passion-week, being times most convenient, both for the temperature of the season and in respect of contagion, which may happen in this near access to his majesty's sacred person. And when his majesty shall at any time think fit to go any progress, he will be pleased to appoint such other times for healing as shall be most convenient. And his majesty doth hereby accordingly order and command, that, from the time of publishing this his majesty's order, none presume to repair to his majesty's court to be healed of the said disease, but only at or within the times for that purpose hereby appointed as aforesaid." Then follow orders for certificates under hand and seal from the vicar, parson or minister, churchwarden, &c., of the parishes of the applicants testifying as to whether they had ever been touched before. Registers were also directed to be kept of these certificates to prevent imposture, and this order was commanded to be read publicly in all parish churches, and then and there affixed to some conspicuous place.

The London Gazette, No. 2180, October

7-11, 1686, contains an advertisement stating that his majesty would heal weekly for the evil upon Fridays, and commanding the attendance of the king's physicians and surgeons at the Meuse upon Thursdays, in the afternoon, to examine the cases and deliver tickets.

The eagerness to obtain certificates from the surgeon was so great, that in Evelyn's 'Diary,' for March 28th, 1684, it is said, "There was so great a concourse of people with their children to be touch'd for the evil, that six or seven were crush'd to death by pressing at the chirurgeon's doore for tickets." (v. i., p. 571.) The number of cases after the restoration appears to have increased greatly, as many as six hundred at a time being touched, and the days appointed being sometimes thrice a week. Some were immediately relieved, others gradually so, and few are reported as not benefited by the practice. The operation was usually performed at Whitehall upon Sundays, and the success attending it may be judged of by the following curious avowal of the king's surgeon: "When I consider his majesties gracious touch, I find myself readily *nonplust*, and shall ever affirm, that all chirurgeons whatsoever must truckle to the same, and come short of his marvellous and miraculous method of healing; and for further manifestation hereof, I do humbly presume to assert, that more souls have been healed by his majesties sacred hand in one year, than have ever been cured by all the physicians and chirurgeons of his three kingdoms ever since his happy restoration. Whereas, should an usurper or tyrant surreptitiously, by pride and bloody massacre, forcibly enter his royal throne and touch at the same experiment, you'll never see such happy success; as tryed by the late usurper *Cromwell* in the late rebellious times; influences flow from thence, he having no more right to the healing power than he had to the royal jurisdiction; his tryal rather chequering and darkening the bright rays hereof and so bringing it into obscurity, than affording it any appearance of light."

Serjeant-Surgeon Wiseman, one of the best early English writers upon surgery, bears testimony to the efficacy of the king's touch, and he devotes an entire book to the subject. He strongly contends for the priority of the English kings over those of France in this matter, and he alludes to the controversy of the time of Edward the Confessor, in which it was disputed whether the cure of the evil were a peculiar reward of the king's holiness, or rather a hereditary faculty attending the English crown. Harpsfield, a renowned divine of the Romish persuasion, describes, in his 'Ecclesiastical History of England,' a miracle wrought by the Confessor, and says, " which admirable faculty of curing the struma, he is justly believed to have transmitted to his posterity, the kings of England, and to have continued it amongst them to those times in which he wrote."*

* " Quam Strumosos sanandi admirabilem dotem in posteros suos Anglorum Reges, ad nostra usque tempora transfudisse et perpetuasse, meritò creditur." (Hist. Anglicana Ecclesiastica, Duaci, 1622, fol. p. 219.

Wiseman says, "I myself have been a frequent eye-witness of many hundreds of cures performed by his majesties' touch alone, without any assistance of chirurgery; and those, many of them, such as had tyred out the endeavours of able chirurgeons before they came thither. It were endless to recite what I myself have seen, and what I have received acknowledgments of by letter, not only from the several parts of this nation, but also from Ireland, Scotland, Jersey, and Guernsey." And he adds, "I must needs profess that what I write will do little more than show the weakness of our ability when compared with his majesty's, who cureth more in any one year than all the chirurgeons of London have done in an age." He points out the cases to which tickets were given for the royal touch. They were to such as have tumours about the neck, and even those accompanied with thick chapped upper lips and eyes affected with a lippitudo.

The king must have suffered no little inconvenience by his possession of the miraculous power; not only was he doomed to those frequent regular days for the healings, private meetings were also held, and Mr. Browne mentions instances in which he alone waited. The king was also beset in his walks by the importunities of the diseased. A most disagreeable case of this kind is reported, upon the authority of the celebrated Elias Ashmole, of a man called Arrice Evans, generally known by the name of Evans, the Prophet, whose condition was so bad that no one could be found willing to recommend him to the sovereign's assistance. He therefore placed himself in St. James's Park, where he knew the king would walk, and upon his majesty's approach called out and attracted the king's notice. Falling down upon his knees, he loudly exclaimed "God bless your majesty!" which occasioned the king to give him his hand to kiss, when Evans availed himself of the opportunity to apply it to his dreadfully ulcerated nose, which from that time improved and ultimately recovered.

It has been remarked as singular, that among the vulgar errors exposed by Sir Thomas Browne, in his 'Pseudodoxia Epidemica,' there should be no mention made of the royal gift of healing; but from a case related in the 'Adenochoiradelogia,' it would seem that this eccentric but able man (who it will be recollected received the honour of knighthood from Charles II) had himself faith in the touch, inasmuch as he recommended the child of a nonconformist in Norfolk, who had been long under his care without receiving benefit, to be taken to the king, then at Breda, or Bruges. Little faith, however, being held by the father of the child as to the efficacy of such intervention, he scorned the advice, and the child was, therefore, under the pretence of a change of air, taken without the privity of the father abroad to the king, where it was submitted to the royal touch and returned perfectly healed. Astonished at the change effected in his child's appearance, the father inquired as to the means that had been employed, and upon being made acquainted with them, he not only acquired faith as to the power of the royal touch, but also cast off his nonconformity; exclaiming, "Farewell to all dissenters and to all nonconformists. If God can put so much virtue into the king's hand so to heal my child, I'll serve that God and that king so long as I live and with all thankfulness."

Mr. Wilkin, in the life of Sir Thomas Browne, prefixed to the edition of his works, published in 1836, in four vols. 8vo., thinks the belief of Sir Thomas Browne in the efficacy of the royal touch to be asserted upon slender grounds; and remarks, that the account given by John Browne, in his 'Adenochoiradelogia,' was after the death of Sir Thomas Browne. I see no reason to question the veracity of the surgeon, as the statement is supported by letters addressed by Sir Thomas Browne to his son, Dr. Edward Browne, and printed by Mr. Wilkin, in one of which, of the date of May 29th, 1679, he says, "Mrs. Verdon went to London to have her sonne touched; if you see her, remember my services;" in another, Oct. 2d, 1679, " His majestie commeth this day to Newmarket; and I shall have occasion to write unto Serjeant Knight, and send certificates for the evill for divers;" in a third, Sept. 22d, 1680, "The king is at Newmarket, and hath good wether for his races and falconrie; divers go from hence to bee touched, butt what chirurgeons are there, I yett understand not, nor what physitians attend his majestie;" and in a fourth, June 6th, 1681, "My cosen Astley his lady went about a fortnight past, and caryed her sonne agayne to Windsor to bee touched agayne, and so he was." Had Sir Thomas Browne regarded the practice as superstitious he would surely, in private letters to his son, who it must be remembered was also a physician, have accompanied these notices with some objurgatory remarks.

Belief in the efficacy of the royal touch for the cure of scrofulous complaints was very general, not only among the ignorant and humble, but with the rich and the educated. It is impossible satisfactorily to account for the credulity of mankind in relation to the cure of diseases; and there are not wanting instances in our own days of reliance upon means the most absurd for the removal of inveterate and incurable disorders. Not only were these marvellous healings wrought by the king through the instrumentality of his touch and the present of the angel gold, but it also appears that the blood of the sacred martyr, Charles I, was equally potent in restoring the sick to health. Wiseman refers to the miracles performed by the blood of his majesty shed upon his decollation by the regicides. Drops of blood were gathered on chips and in handkerchiefs by the pious devotees, who could not but think so great a suffering in so honourable and pious a cause, would be attended by an extraordinary assistance of God and some more than ordinary miracles; nor did their faith, says he, deceive them in this point, there being so many hundreds that found the benefit of it. John Browne also relates several instances of this kind, vouched for by persons in high stations of life, some of whom are at this day known to us by their writings and talent.

From the 'Collection of State Trials'* we learn that in the 36th Charles II, A.D. 1684, Thomas Rosewell, a dissenting teacher, was tried in the Court of King's Bench for high treason; and among other things preferred against him in the indictment were words to the following effect: "That the people made a flocking to the king, upon pretence of healing the king's evil, which he could not do; but we are they to whom they ought to flock, because we are priests and prophets, who can heal their griefs. We have now had two wicked kings together, who have permitted Popery to enter under their noses, whom we can resemble to no other person but to the most wicked Jeroboam: and if you will stand to your principles, I do not fear but we shall be able to overcome our enemies, as in former times, with ramshorns, broken platters, and a stone in a sling. These words three witnesses swore to his having used in a discourse delivered at a conventicle; and, although their testimony was not only unsupported, but distinctly contradicted, the bitterness of the presiding judge (Jefferies) against conventicles and unlicensed preaching was such that it was received, and the prisoner found guilty. He was, however, afterwards pardoned by the king.

JAMES II. This king practised the touch. In the 'Diary of Bishop Cartwright,' lately

---

* Vol. x., p. 147-307.

published, under the editorship of the Rev. Joseph Hunter, by the Camden Society, at the date of August 28, 1687, we read: "I was at his majesty's levee; from whence, at nine o'clock, I attended him into the choir, where he healed 350 persons. After which he went to his devotions in the shire-hall, and Mr. Penn held forth in the tennis-court, and I preached in the Cathedral.* Mr. Creech, in a letter to Dr. Charlett,† says: " On Sunday morning the king (James II) touched, Warner and White officiating; all that waited on his majesty kneeled at the prayers, beside the Duke of Beaufort, who stood all the time."

ANNE. The form of prayer for healing is, as already said, to be found in the 'Book of Common Prayer,' printed in this queen's reign. She touched for the evil at Oxford† and elsewhere. On March 30, 1714, she touched 200 persons, among whom was our celebrated lexicographer and moralist, Dr. Samuel Johnson. He, when four years and half old, was sent to the queen to undergo this ceremony at the instigation of Sir John Floyer, a physician of eminence, who practised at Litchfield, the place of Johnson's birth. Its inefficacy, in this instance at least, was fully established, for he suffered much from the disease during the whole of his life, and bore evidence to the virulence of the disorder.

* The Diary of Dr. Thomas Cartwright, Bishop of Chester. Lond. 1843, 4to., p. 74.
† Aubrey's Letters, vol. i., p. 46.
‡ See Barrington on the Statutes.

Dr. Daniel Turner* relates several cases of scrofula, which had been unsuccessfully treated by himself and Mr. Charles Bernard, serjeant-surgeon to her majesty, yielding afterwards to the efficacy of the royal touch of Queen Anne. "Albeit," says he, "it is the misfortune of some to miss of their cures, after much pain and great expense, yet it has been the good hap of others to obtain one (a cure) in this particular disease, with as little of either (expense or pain); I mean by the *royal touch.*"

Oldmixon† says, "Yesterday the queen was graciously pleased to touch for the king's evil some particular persons in private; and three weeks after, December 19th, yesterday, about twelve at noon, her majesty was pleased to touch at St. James's about twenty persons afflicted with the king's evil. The more ludicrous sort of skeptic's in this case, asked why it was not called the queen's evil, as the chief court of justice was called the Queen's Bench. But Charles Bernard, the surgeon, who had made this touching the subject of his raillery all his lifetime, till he became body surgeon at court, and found it a good perquisite, solved all difficulties by telling his companions with a fleer, '*Really one could not have thought it, if one had not seen it.*' A friend of mine heard him say it, and knew well his opinion of it."

"*Bath*, October 6, a great number of persons coming to this place to be touched by the queen's

---

* Art of Surgery. Lond. 1732, 2 vols., 8vo.
† History of England, vol. ii., p. 302.

majesty for the evil, her majesty commanded Dr. Thomas Gardiner, her chief surgeon, to examine them all particularly, which accordingly was done by him; of whom but thirty appeared to have the evil, which he certified by tickets, as is usual, and those thirty were all touched that day privately, by reason of her majesty's not having a proper conveniency for the solemnity."

The PRETENDERS. Pinkerton's reference to the touch-pieces of the Pretenders seems to warrant the inference that they also attempted to exercise the ceremony of healing. Carte, the historian, was deprived of his annual subsidy from the chamber of London, for asserting the power of healing by the imposition of hands to exist in the Stuart family. This subsidy consisted of a subscription by the corporation of London towards the publication of a History of England. It was unanimously withdrawn in 1748, upon a motion made and seconded by Sir William Calvert and Sir John Barnard; and the work, in consequence, fell into very undeserved neglect. Its merits, however, are correctly appreciated in the present day.

I have thus traced the touching for the evil during the reigns enumerated, in which evidence appears to establish the exercise of the privilege. In reviewing the whole, it is impossible not to feel surprised at the extent of the practice and the length of time that it prevailed. That many persons so touched and labouring under a scrofulous disposition, should receive benefit, may not unfairly be admitted; and an explanation of it is probably afforded by the beneficial effect produced on the system occasioned by the strong feeling of hope and certainty of cure. Such feelings are calculated to impart tone to the system generally, and benefit those of a scrofulous diathesis, in whom the powers are always weak and feeble. According to the extent in which the touching was performed by Charles II, the disease ought, admitting the royal power of healing, to have been exterminated, instead of which we find that during his reign the deaths from the disease exceeded those of any other period. Persons, it must be remembered, flocked from all parts of the country to undergo this operation; and no medical or surgical aid was resorted to.

"Imagination," says Lord Bacon, "is next akin to miracle — a working faith;" and it has been attempted to account for the cures effected by the power of the imagination. There appears, indeed, to be no other natural method to which we can ascribe the good effects recorded on the testimony of Wiseman and other competent authorities. To this, however, it has been objected that infants, who have no apprehension of their case, who can be under no prepossessions, nor capable of exercising any power of fancy, have been as frequently cured as others. Dr. Heylin declares that he has "seen some children brought before the king by the hanging sleeves, some hanging at their mothers' breasts, and others in the arms of their nurses, all touched, and cured without the help of a serviceable imagination."

With the accession of the house of Brunswick the practice of healing by the royal touch ceased.

VALENTINE GREATRAKES' CURES.

About the middle of the seventeenth century, in the reign of Charles II, Mr. Valentine Greatrakes, a gentleman, a member of the Church of England, of great honesty and exemplary sobriety, who is said always to have refused any gratuity for his performances, excited great notoriety, and became, by superstitious feelings, the most celebrated quack of the day. He was a native of Affane, in the county of Waterford, in Ireland, born of a good family, and had received a good education. In 1649, he entered into the service of the English Parliament, and remained in the army until 1656, when, upon the disbandonment of great part of the English, he returned to his native country, and there was engaged in several duties of importance, being registrar for transplantation, a justice of the peace, clerk of the peace for the county of Cork, &c. He lost those places at the time of the Restoration, and it was then, as he describes it, he "felt an impulse that the gift of curing the king's evil was bestowed upon him." His impulse was not long confined to the attempted cure of this solitary disease, for, converts rapidly succeeding, he undertook the cure of ague, epilepsy, convulsions, palsy, deafness, and various other complaints all peculiarly under the influence of the nervous system, and all of which were therefore likely to be benefited by the power exercised over the imagination. He published an account of his cures first in 1666, in the shape of a Letter addressed to the Hon. Robert Boyle, accompanied by testimonials from Bishop Wilkins, Bishop Patrick, Dr. Cudworth, Dr. Whichcot, and others of distinction and intelligence. This book is rare, the greater part of the impression having been destroyed in the great fire of London, and it was not reprinted until 1723, by some one who, believing the cures to have been effected by miraculous and supernatural operation, thought it his duty to revive the subject. Those who may be desirous of examining into the cases, may consult the work already referred to, and 'Stubbe's Miraculous Conformist, or an Account of severall Marvailous Cures performed by the Stroaking of the Hands of Mr. Valentine Greatarick:' Oxford, 1666, 4to.

John Leverett, a gardener, succeeded to the "manual exercise," and declared that, after touching thirty or forty a day, he felt so much goodness go out of him that he was as fatigued as if he had been digging eight roods of ground. This is precisely what is now being affirmed by the animal magnetizers.

SYMPATHETICAL CURES.

> "This is an art
> Which does mend nature ——— but
> The art itself is nature."
>
> WINTER's TALE.

During the reigns of James I and Charles I, a popular belief prevailed in the sympathetical cures of wounds. Sir Kenelm Digby, a gentleman of the bedchamber to Charles I, an eccentric genius, described by Dr. Walter Charleton as "a noble person, who hath built up his reason to so transcendant a height of knowledge, as may seem not much beneath the state of man in innocence," discoursed before an assembly of nobles and learned men at Montpellier in France, "touching the cure of wounds by the powder of sympathy," and professed to have the merit of introducing the same into this quarter of the world. Mr. James Howel, a gentleman celebrated by his 'Dendrologia' and other works, in endeavouring to part two of his friends in a duel, received a severe wound of his hand. Alarmed at this accident, one of the combatants bound up the cut with his garter, took him home, and sent for assistance. The king, upon hearing of the event, sent one of his own surgeons to attend him; but as in the course of four or five days the wound was not recovering very favourably, he made application to Sir Kenelm Digby, of whose knowledge regarding some extraordinary remedies for the healing of wounds he had become apprized. Sir Kenelm first inquired whether he possessed anything that had the blood upon it, upon which Mr. Howel immediately named the garter with which his hand had been bound, which was, accordingly sent for. A basin of water being brought, Sir Kenelm put into it a handful of powder of vitriol, and dissolved it therein. He then took the bloody garter, and immersed it in the fluid, while Mr. H. stood conversing with a gentleman in a corner of the room; but he suddenly started, and, upon being asked the reason, replied that he had lost all pain — that a pleasing kind of freshness, as it were a wet, cold napkin had passed over his hand, and that the inflammation, which before had been so tormenting, had vanished. He was then advised to lay aside all his plasters, to keep the wound clean, and in a moderate temperature. After dinner, the garter was taken out of the basin and placed to dry before a large fire: but no sooner was this done than Mr. H.'s servant came running to Sir Kenelm to say that her master's hand had again inflamed, and that it was as bad as before; whereupon the garter was again placed into the liquid, and before the return of the servant all was well and easy again. In the course of five or six days the wound was cicatrized, and a cure performed.

This case excited considerable attention at

the court, and the king, making inquiry respecting it of Sir Kenelm Digby, his Majesty learnt that the knight had obtained the secret from a Carmelite friar who had travelled in various parts of the world, and who became possessed of it while journeying in the East. Sir Kenelm communicated it to the king's physician, Dr. Mayerne, whence it passed into many hands, so that there was scarce a country barber but had acquaintance with it.

Sir Kenelm Digby's object in his discourse at Montpellier was to show that the sympathetical cure was effected naturally. It would be a waste of time to enter upon a narrative of the eccentric methods employed by Sir Kenelm to explain the action of his powder of sympathy, to detail his conjectures with regard to the emanation of light, the action of the impinging rays, the formation of wind, &c.; but his inferences from these, and his application of them to Mr. Howel's case, may, from his own account, be abridged thus: Mr. Howel received a wound upon his hand — great inflammation followed the injury — his garter was taken covered with the blood from the wound, and steeped in a basin of water in which a quantity of vitriol was dissolved. The basin was kept in the daytime in a closet exposed to the moderate heat of the sun, and at night in the chimney corner, so that the blood upon the garter was always in a good natural temperature. The light of the sun, Sir Kenelm says, will attract from a great extent and distance the spirits of the blood which are upon the garter, and the moderate heat of the hearth will throw off numerous atoms from it. The spirit of vitriol being incorporated with the blood will make the same voyage together with the atoms of the blood. The wounded hand, in the meantime, exhales abundance of hot spirits, which rush forth from the inflamed part, and the wound will consequently draw in the air which is next to it, in the manner of a current, about the wound. With this air is found an incorporation of the atoms of the blood and the vitriol, and those atoms, finding their proper source and original root whence they sprung, remain there in their primitive receptacles, leaving the air to evaporate away. The atoms of the blood and the spirits of vitriol then jointly imbibe together within all the fibres and orifices of the vessels about the wound, which is accordingly comforted, and, in fine, imperceptibly cured. This is, I believe, a fair statement of the opinions of Sir K. Digby and the sympathetical philosophers.*

Their doctrine and the employment of the vitriol is to be traced back to the times of Paracelsus, who, in some points of view, may be considered as the first fabricator of the powder of sympathy. Van Helmont, the panegyrist of his predecessor Paracelsus, acquaints us that the secret was first put forth by Ericcius Mohyus, of Eburo. Van Helmont espoused the doctrine,

* It is very remarkable that, in the Autobiographical Memoir published by Sir Harris Nicholas, from a MS. in the Harleian Collection, Number 6758, Sir Kenelm Digby makes no mention of, or allusion to, the sympathetical cure of wounds.

and extended the practice, combining with it numerous other absurdities in relation to philtres, love potions and powders, sympathies, antipathies, &c. His writings on the 'Magnetick Cure of Wounds,' &c., have been translated by Dr. Charleton, and published under the title of 'A Ternary of Paradoxes,' Lond. 1650, 4to.; and the practice has been supported and defended by Goclenius, Burgravius, Descartes, Kircher, Servius, Baptista Porta, Severinus, Hortmannus, Gilbertus, Papin, Cabæus, Robertus Fludd, &c., &c. Charleton ascribes the cures to magnetism.

The method described by Sir Kenelm Digby in Mr. Howel's case, was that which is called the cure by the wet way; but it was also effected in a dry way; and Straus, in a letter to Sir Kenelm, gives an account of a cure performed by Lord Gilbourne, an English nobleman, upon a carpenter who had cut himself severely with his axe. The axe, bespattered with blood, was sent for, besmeared with an ointment, wrapped up warmly, and carefully hung up in a closet. The carpenter was immediately relieved, and all went on well for some time, when, however, the wound became exceedingly painful, and, upon resorting to his lordship, it was ascertained that the axe had fallen from the nail by which it was suspended, and thereby become uncovered!

Dryden, in the 'Tempest,' Act. v., sc. 1, makes Ariel to say, in reference to the wound received by Hippolito from Ferdinand —

"He must be dress'd again, as I have done it.
Anoint the sword which pierced him with this weapon-salve, and wrap it close from air, till I have time to visit him again."

And in the next scene the following dialogue ensues between Hippolito and Miranda:

Hip. O my wound pains me.
Mir. I am come to ease you.
[She unwraps the sword.
Hip. Alas! I feel the cold air come to me;
My wound shoots worse than ever.
[She wipes and anoints the sword.
Mir. Does it still grieve you?
Hip. Now methinks, there's something
Laid just upon it.
Mir. Do you find no ease?
Hip. Yes, yes, upon the sudden, all the pain
Is leaving me. Sweet heaven, how I am eased!

Werenfels says, "If the superstitious person be wounded by any chance, he applies the salve, not to the wound, but, what is more effectual, to the weapon by which he received it. By a new kind of art, he will transplant his disease, like a scion, and graft it into what tree he pleases."

There is no doubt that the practice was at one time very general, but it would now be a waste of time to go into the particulars respecting the various compositions of the sympathetical curers; the manner in which their vitriol was to be prepared by exposure for 365 days to the sun, the unguents of human fat and blood, mummy, moss of dead man's skull, bull's blood and fat, and other disgusting ingredients; it may, however, be told as characteristic of the ignorance, superstition, and barbarity of the age, that a serious discussion was long maintained in consequence of a schism in the sympathetical school, " whether it was necessary that the moss should grow absolutely in the skull of a thief who had hung on the gallows, and whether the ointment, while compounding, was to be stirred with a murderer's knife?" " You smile," says Van Helmont, " because Goclenius chooses for an ingredient into the unguent that moss only which is gathered off the skull of a man of *three letters*" (F U R).

It is not at all surprising that cures of the description alluded to should soon be looked upon as the result of magic, incantations, and other supernatural means; and that the professors of the sympathetic art, therefore, should have been anxious to account for the effects by natural causes. Such appears to have been Sir Kenelm Digby's chief aim before the doctors of Montpellier, and similar reasonings upon the subject may be found in the writings of the supporters of the system already mentioned, who advocated the plan of treatment and vouched for its efficacy. In this search for natural means to account for the phenomena obtained, the obvious one was overlooked; and the history I have given would be uninteresting but for the valuable practical lesson which these experiments have afforded. We owe to this folly the introduction of one of the first principles of surgery — one which in this country has done more to advance the science than any other beside — one which has saved a vast amount of human suffering and preserved innumerable lives. The history of the doctrine of healing wounds by the powder of sympathy is the history of adhesion — the history of union by the first intention — a history which until the time of John Hunter was never fairly developed or distinctly comprehended.

It has been well observed by the late Mr. John Bell, that "it is an old, but a becoming and modest thought, that in our profession we are but the ministers of nature; and indeed the surgeon, still more than the physician, achieves nothing by his own immediate power, but does all his services by observing and managing the properties of the living body; where the living principle is so strong and active in every part that by that energy alone it regenerates any lost substance, or reunites in a more immediate way the more simple wounds." A wound, in general terms, may be defined to be a breach in the continuity of the soft parts of the body; and an incised wound is the most simple of its kind. These, it must be remembered, were of the description of wounds to which the sympathetical curers resorted, and their secret of cure is to be explained by the rest and quiet which the wounded parts were permitted to enjoy, in opposition to the ordinary treatment under the fallacious doctrine and practice of that day in digesting, mundificating, incarnating, &c. Surgeons in former times seem really by their modes of treatment to have tried how far it was possible to impede instead of to facilitate the processes of nature; and to those who are acquainted with modern surgery it almost appears miraculous that they ever should have been able to have produced union of any wound whatever. What is the mode of treatment now employed by the surgeon in the healing of a wound? To clear it from extraneous matter, to bring the edges in apposition, to keep them in contact by a proper bandage, to modify temperature, and to give rest. What is this but the mode of procedure on the part of the sympathetical curers? They washed the wound with water, kept it clean and undisturbed, and in a few days the union of parts — the process of adhesion — was perfected, and the cure was complete. The doctrine of adhesion, the exudation of lymph, the junction of old or the formation of new vessels, and the consequent agglutination of parts was then ill understood: subtle and, in many instances it must be admitted, ingenious reasons were resorted to, to account for the effects produced, and the true solution of the process was everlooked — the effect was apparent but the cause was obscure.

The rapidity with which a restoration of the continuity of parts is effected is astonishing. It is not at all uncommon to find after operations a union of the severed parts, to a very considerable extent, produced in twenty-four, thirty-six, or forty-eight hours. I have seen the whole surface of an amputated limb healed in the course of three days. The reported cures, therefore, of the sympathetic doctors are easily to be credited, and the mystery connected with it dispelled by the lights of modern surgery and physiology. It is worthy of remark that gunshot wounds never can heal by the adhesive process, and that in no instance does it appear that attempts were made by the sympathists to interfere in these cases. Their operations were judiciously confined to simple incised wounds; and these we have seen are of a description readily to unite if properly cleansed, brought together, and left undisturbed.

The Taliacotian art owes its origin to the doctrine of adhesion; but this forms not any part of the present inquiry, inasmuch as it did not emanate from any preconceived superstition entertained respecting it.

The cruel practices of ancient surgeons are now happily abolished; nature is the guide, and her operations must be watched with scrupulous accuracy. Nothing can give greater satisfaction to the humane surgeon and philosopher than the contemplation of the change of practice resulting from modern researches in the healing art: advantage has been taken of the errors of our ancestors, and their blunders even turned to present good. To dwell upon the subject any longer is unnecessary, as the powers of nature in the restoration of parts is fully established and well understood; and to such an extent does this exist that we know that parts entirely separated from the body have been reapplied and united.* There are not wanting well-au-

* Garengeot, a celebrated French Surgeon, asserts that he had seen a nose which had been bitten off in a quarrel, thrown

thenticated cases of the union of the nose, ear, and other parts of the body, after being nearly

upon the ground, allowed to get cool, taken up, fixed to the face, and adhere again; and he records (Traité des Operations de Chirurgie, vol. iii.), that M. Galin produced a similar union of a considerable portion of the nose after it had been bitten off and spit out into a dirty gutter. It was well washed, and, upon the return of the soldier, who, having suffered this mutilation, had pursued his adversary, re-applied to his face. Garengeot examined the man on the fourth day, and found the wound completely cicatrized. — Blegny (Zodiacus Medico-Gallicus, Mar. 1680) records a similar case of union after a sabre cut; and Mr. Carpue, in his excellent 'Account of Two Successful Operations for restoring a Lost Nose,' makes reference to Lombard, Loubet, and others, who have been successful in like cases. — Sir Leonard Fioravanti, a Bolognese, states, in his 'Rational Secrets and Chirurgery Reviewed,' that, when in Africa, he was witness to a dispute between a Spanish gentleman and a military officer, which led to a combat, in which the latter struck off the nose of his adversary, and it fell into the sand. Fioravanti took it up, washed it with warm water, dressed the part with his balsam, bound it up, and left it undisturbed during eight days, at the expiration of which time he examined it, and was surprised to find that the wounded parts had adhered. — Taliacotius relates that, in a fray between some drunken young men, one of the party had his nose cut off by a sword. The assailant fled, and was pursued by his opponent, regardless of his nose, which was left in a gutter. Taliacotius picked it up, cleaned it, and, upon the return of its owner, adjusted the cut surfaces with particular accuracy, so that complete adhesion followed. — The 'Journal Hebdomadaire' records two cases by Dr. Barthelemy in which union of the nose had taken place after complete separation. One was that of an officer at Lyons, in 1815, who had the end of his nose cut off in a duel by his adversary's sabre. He put the severed portion in his pocket, kept it warm, returned home and sent for a surgeon, who replaced it, and adhesion was effected. The other case, which is given on the authority of Dr. Regnault, was in a man who, in a fight with another, had part of his nose bitten off. He separated from it, hanging by a very small portion of skin, sufficient, however, to support the

wrapped it up in his handkerchief, put it into his pocket, and for four or five hours only bewailed his loss. He was at length urged to apply to a surgeon, who steeped it in warm alcohol, placed the divided parts in contact, and in ten days they were reunited. — Portions of the ear have also been cut off, reapplied, and union effected. I know one case in which the entire ear was torn off, carefully replaced, and perfect adhesion procured. — A case no less extraordinary, perhaps more so, from the structure of the parts concerned, was related in the 'Edinburgh Medical and Surgical Journal' for 1814. It occurred in Scotland, and is judicially attested. A finger was entirely cut off, replaced and united, suffering only the loss of the nail. — Mr. Peacock, a surgeon, at Liverpool, communicated to the editors of the 'London Medical Repository' (vol. vi., p. 368) a case of union of a finger, divided at the middle joint. A young gentleman, about ten years of age, cut through the middle joint of his forefinger with a carving knife so completely, that the part of the finger beyond the division was hanging by a piece of the integument not thicker than a common probe. The ligaments and bloodvessels were completely divided. The severed parts were placed in apposition, and firmly retained by a splint. At the expiration of eight days, the parts had completely united. The natural warmth and sensation of the finger gradually returned, and the motion of the joint became as free and extensive as it had been before the accident. — Garengeot mentions a similar case effected by M. Bossu, a surgeon, at Arras, in which a boy cut off the third phalanx of the thumb of his left hand. He put the severed part into his pocket and went to the surgeon, who washed it in warm wine, reapplied it, and was successful in obtaining complete adhesion. — These, however, not more surprising than the preparations in the Hunterian museum at the Royal College of Surgeons, where a human tooth, upon being extracted, was immediately inserted into the comb of a cock, where it became nourished and remained. This was done by John Hunter. Mr. John Bell disputed the fact, nay, he totally disbelieved it; but, upon visiting the museum one day with Sir Astley Cooper, the preparations upon which he first vitality of the part, and enable it to go through those processes necessary for rendering it again a constituent part of the frame.

fixed his eye were the sections of the cock's head, upon which the baronet good-naturedly observed, "Ah! he does indeed stare you in the face." — The late Mr. Hodgson, a celebrated surgeon at Lewes, when a boy, had his nose so cut that the only bond of union was a small portion of skin by which it hung. His mother replaced the nose, and it united. The cicatrix was visible to the day of his death, which lately occurred at an advanced age. — The 'Journal der Chirurgie und Augen-Heilkunde' (B. 7, H. 4) relates two cases in which the nose was united after a complete separation from the face. In one of these cases, two hours elapsed before the severed part was sought after and applied, but the union was perfectly successful.

THE END.

www.ingramcontent.com/pod-product-compliance
Lightning Source LLC
Chambersburg PA
CBHW062320220526
45469CB00008B/2569